Your Career in Nursing

Sixth Edition

Annette Vallano, MS, RN, APRN, BC

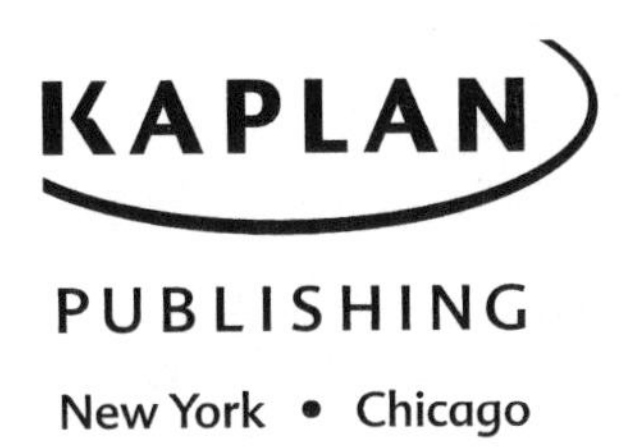

New York • Chicago

NCLEX-RN® is a trademark of the National Council of State Boards of Nursing, which neither sponsors nor endorses this product.

This publication is designed to provide accurate and authoritative information in regard to the subject matter covered. It is sold with the understanding that the publisher is not engaged in rendering legal, accounting, or other professional service. If legal advice or other expert assistance is required, the services of a competent professional should be sought.

© 2011 Annette T. Vallano

Published by Kaplan Publishing, a division of Kaplan, Inc.
395 Hudson Street
New York, NY 10014

All rights reserved. The text of this publication, or any part thereof, may not be reproduced in any manner whatsoever without written permission from the publisher.

Bennett Swingle, Anne. "Still Not Much of a Guy Thing." *Hopkins Medicine* (a publication of the Johns Hopkins Medical Institute). By permission of the author.

Cataldo, Jackie. "Smoke and Debris". Reprinted with permission from the *Journal of the New York State Nurses Association,* Spring/Summer 2002, Volume 33, Number 1.

Shihab Nye, Naomi. "The Art of Disappearing." By permission of the author.

Williams, Michael. "President's Notes: A Journey of Rediscovery: So How Does It Feel to You?" *AACN News,* August 2001. By permission of the author.

Wilson, Bruce, RN, PhD "Men in American Nursing History," *www.geocities.com/~brucewilson*. By permission of the author.

"Nursing. It's real. It's life." Courtesy of Nurses for a Healthier Tomorrow.

"Be a Nurse." Courtesy of Johnson & Johnson Services, Inc., The Campaign for Nursing's Future.

Printed in the United States of America

Library of Congress Cataloging-in-Publication Data

Vallano, Annette.
Your career in nursing : managing your future in the changing world of healthcare / Annette Vallano.—6th ed.
p. ; cm.
Includes bibliographical references and index.
ISBN 978-1-4277-9787-2 (pbk. : alk. paper)
1. Nursing—Vocational guidance. I. Title.
[DNLM: 1. Nursing. 2. Career Choice. 3. Professional Competence. 4. Vocational Guidance. WY 16 V177y 2008]

RT82.V34 2008
610.730699—dc22 2008035883

10 9 8 7 6 5 4 3 2 1

ISBN-13: 978-1-60714-834-0

Kaplan Publishing books are available at special quantity discounts to use for sales promotions, employee premiums, or educational purposes. For more information or to purchase books, please call the Simon & Schuster special sales department at 866-506-1949.

Your Career in Nursing

Other Kaplan Books for Nurses

NCLEX-RN®: Strategies for the Registered Nurse Licensing Exam
NCLEX-PN®: Strategies for the Practical Nursing Licensing Exam
NCLEX-RN®: Medications You Need to Know for the Exam

How to Survive Clinical
First Year Nurse
Kaplan Legal Nurse Certification
Kaplan CCRN

Medical Terms for Nurses
Spanish for Nurses
Math for Nurses

Home Delivery: A Midwife's Journey Through Motherhood and Other Miracles

Kaplan Voices: Nurses
Reflections on Doctors: Nurses' Stories about Physicians and Surgeons
Meditations on Hope: Nurses' Stories about Motivation and Inspiration
Final Moments: Nurses' Stories about Death and Dying

Saving Lives: Why the Media's Portrayal of Nurses Puts Us All at Risk

The End-of-Life Advisor: Personal, Legal, and Medical Considerations for a Peaceful, Dignified Death

TABLE OF CONTENTS

PART ONE: Today's Healthcare Landscape

PART TWO: Converting Your Nursing Career into *You, Inc.*

Appendix

ABOUT THE AUTHOR

Annette T. Vallano, MS, RN, APRN, BC, is a board-certified clinical nurse specialist and psychoanalyst in private practice in New York City. Her long-standing interest in the professional and personal well-being of nurses has shaped her career for more than 25 years and continues to occupy an important place in her work.

Annette has transformed her nursing career many times. A diploma graduate of St. John's Episcopal Hospital in Brooklyn, New York, she went on to receive her BSN and MS from Adelphi University. She has been a direct care nurse in pediatrics and obstetrics; an army nurse; a nurse manager; a nurse educator; a consultant and entrepreneur; a career coach; a nurse psychotherapist; and now a psychoanalyst following the completion of her studies at the Institute for Contemporary Psychotherapy in New York City where she is a member of the Training Committee, which coordinates the learning experience of and advocates for candidates in psychoanalytic training.

Considering herself a learner, seeker, and perpetual student, Annette is currently studying eating disorders with an interest in developing a model of managing obesity and compulsive overeating that integrates both psychological and physical experiences.

She is a seeker of work-life balance with interests in fine dining, ballroom dancing, and ocean cruising. Annette's extensive experience as an employed and self-employed nurse give her firsthand knowledge of the complexities, challenges, and amazing rewards of nursing practice.

CONTRIBUTORS

Karen A. Ballard, MA, RN, FAAN, is a nurse consultant in private practice specializing in professional practice issues and the development of health policy. She has her bachelor's degree in nursing from Niagra University and her master's degree in child and adolescent psychiatric–mental health nursing from New York University. Ms. Ballard is a consultant to The Luminary Project of Health Care Without Harm, an international coalition of 450 organizations in 54 countries working to make the healthcare industry environmentally responsible. She is also an adjunct faculty member in PACE University's Lienhard School of Nursing, lecturing on psychiatric–mental health nursing and professional nursing issues. For the previous 20 years, Ms. Ballard held various staff positions with the New York State Nurses Association, including director of special projects and director of the Practice and Governmental Affairs Program, where she interpreted nursing practice issues; served as a lobbyist; and addressed such issues as bioterrorism, HIV/AIDS, reimbursement, nursing acuity, and the nursing shortage. She is the President (2009–2011) of the New York State Nurses Association and the First Vice-President (2010–2012) of the American Nurses Association. Her recent publications include the textbook *Psychiatric–Mental Health Nursing—An Introduction to Theory and*

Practice and articles on environmental health nursing in various nursing publications. She authored chapter 2 of this book: "Nursing Practice."

David N. Ekstrom, PhD, RN, is an Associate Professor and the Director of Student International Affairs at the Lienhard School of Nursing, Pace University, New York, where he has taught for over 15 years. Dr. Ekstrom holds a bachelor's degree in biology from Oberlin College, a bachelor's degree in nursing from Columbia University, and both master's and PhD degrees in nursing from New York University, where his doctoral dissertation, "Gender and Perceived Nurse Caring in Nurse-Patient Dyads," won the NYU Women's Studies Award for excellence in feminist research. At Pace, Dr. Ekstrom teaches in both the undergraduate and graduate programs, focusing on professional issues, culture and diversity, nursing theory, and comparative healthcare systems. He has published and presented on diverse topics, including online education in nursing, international experiences in nursing education, and fathers of children with special needs.

Dr. Marilyn Jaffe-Ruiz, EdD, MEd, MA, is a professor of nursing at the Lienhard School of Nursing, Pace University. Her specialties are nursing education, psychiatric mental health nursing, communication, cultural diversity, and leadership. Dr. Jaffe-Ruiz was Pace University's Chief Academic Officer from 1994 to 2004 with the title of Provost and Executive Vice President for Academic Affairs from 1998 to 2003, until her return to being a professor of nursing in 2004. Formerly, she was Vice Provost and, prior to that, Dean of the Lienhard School of Nursing. She has had extensive experience in psychiatric/ mental health nursing, including as a private practitioner.

Dr. Jaffe-Ruiz has chaired the Task Force on Diversity, lectured on managing cultural diversity in the workforce, and consulted on cultural diversity in healthcare.

She was inducted into the Teachers College Nursing Hall of Fame by the Teachers College Nursing Educational Alumni Association and made an honorary member of the Golden Key International Honor Society at Pace University. In 2002, she received the Diversity Leadership Award at Pace University. Dr. Jaffe-Ruiz received the University's Diversity Leadership Award in 2002 and the Martin Luther King Social Justice Award in 2006.

William R. Donovan, MA, RN, has a BS in nursing from Adelphi University and an MA in nursing from New York University. He is a systems analyst in the information technology department at The Mount Sinai Hospital in New York City.

He has given many lectures and received several awards for his nursing work and holds a Six Sigma green belt. He has served on many nursing organizational committees, most recently completing a four-year elected term on the American Nurses Association Congress on Nursing Practice and Economics. He recently completed a term as treasurer for Nurses House, Inc. and currently serves as a board member on the Nurses House board.

PREFACE

There has never been a better time to be a nurse or to consider nursing as a career. The nursing shortage, the influence of managed care, and the use of technology are reshaping the healthcare landscape and filling its many workplaces with opportunities and challenges for all those willing to embrace change.

In writing this book, I hope you will find the information and support you will need to make intelligent choices about your career and to feel invigorated about how you can work and what you can offer. Every nurse across all generations, genders, and cultures has a sphere of influence from which to make a unique contribution. This might be your nursing skills and competencies, your proficiency with technology, your ability to teach, your creative problem solving, your political activism, or any of the other talents and abilities I know you have. Opportunities abound, and each segment of the nursing profession has something important to contribute:

> **The newly graduated nurse** contributes a contagious infusion of new energy and bright idealism, as well as a desire to learn that enlivens all those with whom he or she comes in contact, whether patient, coworker, or colleague.
>
> **The second-career nurse** brings invaluable maturity and enthusiasm in the achievement of a long-sought goal, along with a fresh perspective that draws on valuable prior work and life experience.
>
> **Men who become nurses** bring an important dynamic of balance to this too-long female-dominated profession, challenging us to strive for better gender diversity while reminding us that caring, compassion, and intelligence are gender-neutral characteristics.
>
> **The mature nurse** represents the "brain trust" of our profession and passes down this knowledge and wisdom, whether in the role of coworker, preceptor, mentor, or coach. An unexpected contribution of the mature nurse, which may benefit all nurses, is the improvement of workplace policies and ergonomics as employers seek to retain this nurse in order to ease the nursing shortage.

Now more than ever, being a nurse requires information, insight, and resilience. I've worked side by side with you for many years, in many capacities. I know the obstacles you face, and I know your ability to transform these obstacles into challenges and to conquer them.

I honor and support the depth of your caring and the strength of your power. I hope you will use the winds of change to set sail in the direction of making your voice heard and your actions matter. I'm so proud to work among you!

DEDICATION

To those who surrounded, protected, and ministered to me, taking turns, each in their own way standing guard at the gates of hell during those unexpected and difficult days in 2009:

TO CAROL:

You lived as a New Yorker again, foregoing Florida sunshine to stand against the darkness while you protected, advocated, and encouraged. ***Thank you.***

TO KAREN:

You, along with Carol, made essential decisions and coordinated resources when I couldn't, even about the *Nutcracker*! ***Thank you.***

TO BARBARA:

My BBF (Best Buddy Forever), your daily calls were a loving and healing lifeline: Zalewski would have approved! ***Thank you.***

TO PHYLLIS:

Sisters always, through thick and thin; you were just as present on the phone as you would have been in person . . . the miles never separated us. ***Thank you.***

TO JUDITH:

You held onto what you knew my life to be when I was unable to remember. ***Thank you.***

And especially to the nurses and nursing staff of 6 West at The Mount Sinai Hospital, New York City, and the Emergency Department Staff of The Allen Pavilion, New York Presbyterian Hospital, New York City:

"*Your* Careers in Nursing" are appreciated by me in ways that words can never fully express. Each of you contributed to my well-being and recovery. I am proud to call you colleagues and count myself among you. ***Thank you.***

PART ONE

Today's Healthcare Landscape

CHAPTER 1

Today's Nurse

We live in a time of rapid change and contradictory realities. We have inherited the 20th century's excesses and jolting changes while finding ourselves on a collision course with the 21st century's fantastic forecasts and harsh awakenings. For those of us who are nurses, this translates into the often contradictory realities of patient care and managed care; the ubiquitous challenge of ever-changing technology in the healthcare arena; the harsh awakening of the nursing shortage; and the fantastic forecasts of such medical advances as genomics, regenerative medicine, and robotic surgery.

> It was the best of times, it was the worst of times,
>
> It was the age of wisdom, it was the age of foolishness,
>
> It was the epoch of belief, it was the epoch of incredulity,
>
> It was the season of light, it was the season of darkness,
>
> It was the spring of hope, it was the winter of despair,
>
> We had everything before us, we had nothing before us,
>
> We were all going direct to heaven, we were all going direct the other way.
>
> —*Charles Dickens, A Tale of Two Cities*[1]

THE EARTH AS A GLOBAL VILLAGE

The proliferation of information technologies and personal computers in the late 20th century has fulfilled its promise of creating closer global relationships by shrinking the world into what is now commonly called a "global village". We are in the midst of a continuing paradigm shift in which countries, companies, and individuals are learning to communicate and compete in a global marketplace. We live in the dual reality of people losing jobs to offshore locations while simultaneously benefiting from resources and services not easily available otherwise. Dial a U.S. phone number for tech support if you have a glitch in your latest technology purchase, and you are just as likely to be linked with a person from India or Ireland as one from the United States.

The potentially apocalyptic impact of climate change emerged out of what could be called the 20th century's "season of darkness," a time of excess and apparent inability or unwillingness to understand the human impact on the planet. Our "spring of hope" may come in the form of the 21st century's "green revolution," which aims to propel the world into a brighter future through the work of increasingly enlightened companies, entrepreneurial enthusiasm, and the development of sustainable products and policies.

THE BEST AND WORST OF TIMES IN HEALTHCARE

That the healthcare industry is within the grip of its best and worst of times seems evident. For example:

- We are inevitably drawn to the convenience and ease of computer technology and the Internet, while simultaneously becoming overloaded by the demands that it places on our lives as well as concerned about protecting our privacy. For example, for many of us, the idea of storing our health records on Web-based healthcare sites conjures up both relief over ease of access and anxiety over a potential lack of privacy.
- The promise of medical science's elaborate new treatments, some of which can be tailored to personalized genetic profiles, seems to fly in the face of our ability to solve the grave dilemma and fallout of the nation's 47 million uninsured or underinsured people.[2] We have the best of medical science, but it's only available to those who can afford it.
- While nurses are poised to benefit from the promising forecast of excellent job growth and opportunity on one hand, they also find themselves faced with large workloads and concerns about being able to provide safe patient care as a result of a nursing shortage. Just as uncertainty accompanies so many complex issues in these early years of the 21st century, it is also present when attempting to predict the outcome of the nursing shortage. Two factors that could lessen the impact of this shortfall of nurses are an economic recession, in which more nurses would need to work, and/or the delayed retirement of the baby boom generation of nurses. For more discussion of these issues, see chapters 2 and 6.

The Dickens quote that opens this chapter begins his well-known story of the French Revolution. To use it in a discussion of the current healthcare revolution is apt—the antecedents of both revolutions are similar with regard to the levels of social unrest and frustration that preceded each of them.

A revolution is an attempt to overthrow or renounce current unsound circumstances. In France, these circumstances were the political and social systems that created inequality among the citizens, favoring the nobility and clergy above the bourgeoisie, who at that time were merchants and traders. Likewise, a kind of caste system exists within today's healthcare industry, blocking access to services for large segments of the population.

Just as the French people revolted and took destiny into their own hands, so too do we find a corollary within the current healthcare revolution. Consider the emergence of targeted, consumer-friendly healthcare sites, often staffed by nurse practitioners offering nonemergency care in such retail centers as Wal-Mart. These so-called quick-clinics, sometimes nicknamed "McMedical Care," provide the fast, convenient, and less costly care Americans have been unable to find within traditional healthcare settings.

THE HEALTHCARE REVOLUTION MARCHES ON

The Recent Past: The Late 20th Century

Most would place the beginning of the current healthcare revolution in the 1990s, when social, political, and economic factors led to the onset of managed care with its fiscal restraint and cost containment. There was a growing awareness that the U.S. healthcare system was broken, that there was no organized system of healthcare but rather an increasingly costly system of disease care. Managed care emerged in response to this fractured system and developed methods of oversight that capped payments to healthcare providers with the goal of reducing costs.

This led to the era of downsizing and organizational restructuring. Job security was threatened for millions, especially nurses, for the first time in the history of our profession. However, despite the surplus of nurses created by the economic necessities of downsizing, a simultaneous nursing shortage was predicted to grow more severe as the demand for nurses outstripped the supply of qualified nurses willing to work. Whatever shape the current nursing shortage cycle takes, it is sure to impact the practicing nurse today as well as to influence the quality of patient care. Information about the nursing shortage is woven in throughout this book, particularly in chapters 2 and 3.

On the Edge of Transformation: The Early 21st Century

The 21st century challenges us with its complex realities and possibilities. The changes we are experiencing require shifts in thinking, working, and living. It is essential to be ready to adapt and to embrace these changes. Of all the skills required of today's nurse, the ability to adapt to cycles of rapid, complex change is as vital as any clinical skill you can name. The capacity to become change-hardy and resilient enables you to go beyond just surviving these times to thriving and benefitting from them. We will explore the topic of managing change in chapter 15.

Current Healthcare Trends

The following summary represents a small sampling of what is happening now and what may be just around the corner. Nurses who want successful 21st-century careers need to track these and other trends to prepare for changing roles and to take advantage of new career options.

Technology is a megatrend, and it's everywhere! No longer new or novel, technology, including personal and networked computers, the Internet, and intranets, has become a vital part of healthcare operations and an integral component of patient care. Personal digital assistants (PDAs) are loaded with textbooks. Computer terminals store **electronic medical records (EMRs),** allowing every member of the healthcare team to access the same information remotely. Technology is so ubiquitous that it could easily be considered another member of the clinical or management team! We are long past the time when nurses had an option about their computer literacy. Technology is not only changing how nurses work but how they learn, as evidenced by the multiplying **online learning** venues for basic, graduate, and ongoing nursing education.

Additional trends in technology include the expanding use of **telemedicine** and **telenursing,** especially for the **remote monitoring of patients** at home or even in ICUs, and the potentially controversial implementation of the **portable electronic medical record** with its privacy issues yet to be solved. Career options for nurses interested in healthcare technology include **nursing informatics** and consulting roles during the design and implementation of such programs as **telenursing** or **EMRs.** For more about technology, refer to chapter 4.

Advances in medical science will include the use of **genomics** and **pharmacogenomics**, with targeted treatment options developed through the use of a patient's own DNA; **regenerative medicine,** which creates living, functional tissues to repair or replace damaged tissue or organs; and the use of **robotics** in surgical procedures.

The **globalization of healthcare** will result in the utilization of a worldwide labor force to purchase healthcare products and services beyond a country's borders. This will allow access to products and services that may be less costly or more available, such as technology-related services.

The **commodization of healthcare** will result in healthcare clinics (often staffed by nurse practitioners) in retail centers. These are emerging rapidly to satisfy consumers' desires for services of lower cost, greater convenience, and easier accessibility. They are especially attractive to people with limited or no health insurance.

Cost containment will continue to be a prominent influence in how healthcare services are delivered, as prices are fueled by inflation and increasing demand. Coupled with the significant labor shortages predicted, the idea of "do more with less" is not going away anytime soon. For nurses, this issue is crucial to quality patient care and just as crucial to the quality of work-life balance. The necessity of developing a self-care practice when working in this type of challenging environment will be discussed further in chapter 15.

The **health insurance crisis,** with 47 million Americans uninsured and underinsured (U.S. Census Bureau 2007),[2] will continue to require creative problem solving for healthcare organizations faced with how to care for these patients who wind up in their emergency rooms.

Pay-For-Performance (P4P) is a reimbursement model based on quality patient indicators, some tied to medical outcomes and others to nursing care, such as catheter-associated urinary track infections and pressure ulcers. Poised to be implemented by the Centers for Medicare and Medicaid Services in October 2008, P4P is being watched closely to ensure that the increased scrutiny of nursing care is used to identify nursing's critical role in effective and safe patient care rather than to blame an understaffed nursing workforce for untoward complications resulting from the current nursing shortage. To understand more about the pros and cons of this important issue, read "Wrestling with a New Reality" by Barbara Kirshheimer (Nursing Spectrum 7/14/08) or log on to *www.nurse.com* or *www.nursingworld.org*.[3]

The **aging baby boom generation** is anticipated to influence healthcare organizations greatly. Not only is this age cohort expected to create a tidal wave of health needs, but its exit from the healthcare workforce will also be keenly felt. In chapter 6, you'll find a broader discussion of issues related to retaining mature nurse in the healthcare workforce.

As you will read in chapter 2, the current **nursing shortage** has lasted longer than any shortage since the 1960s and is expected to continue well into the 21st century. While the current shortage is driven by several factors, including an aging population of nurses and fewer younger people entering the workforce, important mitigating circumstances also should be watched carefully. They include what direction the national economy takes, because difficult financial times are likely to keep more nurses in the workforce. Another important influence on the shortage will be the ergonomic and policy changes healthcare employers are beginning to make in an effort to meet the needs of the mature nurse. How this is anticipated to benefit all employed nurses, as well as how the four generations of nurses working today are influencing nursing practice, will be discussed in chapter 6.

Look for the disease management model of healthcare, also called case management or care coordination, to morph into models of **population-based healthcare**. Shifting to a population-based system extends strategies of disease management to large groups, such as health plan enrollees with specific diagnoses (diabetes, for example). Wellness programs offered by employers, such as smoking cessation, are another example of population-based care. This area is expected to continue to offer many interesting career opportunities for nurses.

There will be an increasing focus on **evidence-based practice (EBP)** in which nurses integrate current research and expert opinions on clinical practice into their own nursing practice, whether as direct care nurses, administrators, educators, or researchers. Chapters 2 and 4 contain additional discussions about this important trend. Seeking out employment where EBP is utilized is important for your professional development and a smart career move as well.

With two-thirds of Americans significantly overweight or obese, a cultural shift is sweeping the country. Some healthcare experts, including the Centers for Disease Control and Prevention, believe that as obesity and its related health issues rises, it will compete with tobacco as the leading preventable cause of death (JAMA 2004).[4] Targeting **obesity as a public health crisis** and "epidemic" will generate wellness and weight loss programs aimed at facilitating healthy lifestyles. Nurses have excellent opportunities to be at the forefront of this issue, given their focus on primary prevention, nutrition, and education. Look for career opportunities in centers offering bariatric surgery as well as obesity/weight management-related services.

Environmental issues have always been a concern for nurses. Florence Nightingale and many others who followed her have long since correlated human health and recovery from illness with environmental conditions. The **Green Revolution**, with its mushrooming array of sustainable policies and products, extends these ideas. Watch for the continued development and reliance on environmentally friendly operating practices and building construction guidelines for healthcare facilities. **Health Care Without Harm** is an international coalition of over 473 organizations in 50 countries whose mission is to "transform the healthcare sector worldwide, without compromising patient safety or care, so that it is ecologically sustainable and no longer a source of harm to public health and the environment." You can track such issues as green purchasing, healthy building, and mercury disposal at *www.noharm.org*.

This area is fertile with career options for nurses with vision and creativity in the use of their nursing knowledge and expertise. Such a nurse is Karen Ballard, the contributing author of chapter 2, who consults for Health Care Without Harm. For inspiring stories about nurses who are already incorporating environmental health into their nursing practice, go to *www.theluminaryproject.org*.

REALIGNING OUR VALUES

We are indeed living in a world hard to imagine only a short time ago. Horrific tragedies, including the 2008 earthquake in China and cyclone in Myanmar, the 2010 earthquake in Haiti, the continuing war in Iraq, and the threat of worldwide terrorism, continue to change our world and how we live in it. Add to this the potentially apocalyptic effects of climate change, with its evidence of how humans have impacted the planet over the last 50 years, and we find ourselves grappling with questions of freedom and responsibility and asking how civilized people are supposed to behave and respond.

Many of us are rethinking our values, our priorities, the meaning we want our lives to have, and the way in which we want to spend our time. We are more keenly aware of the unpredictability of life and are taking a second look at the quality of our careers, our work lives, and our relationships. Rhema Ellis,[5] a reporter for NBC News, summarized the essence of this reevaluation after she interviewed a cross section of the nation's 2002 graduating classes:

> Graduates are asking themselves, "How can I help?" rather than "What do I want?" They are less preoccupied with indulgence and more focused on reflection; they are feeling a greater responsibility for making a contribution to the world. Many are more interested in employment in the nonprofit world than in corporate America. There is a shift in predominant life values as reflected in a concern with what one does in one's life rather than what one has. Many are

> expressing a desire to make a difference, to do more than just have a job. Whether or not the graduate has changed their career path as a result of 9/11, most have committed themselves to be more effective in their daily life.

Many of the values, desires, and concerns expressed by these graduates will continue to ring true, and they have always been inherent in the profession of nursing. The desire "to make a difference, to do more than just have a job" is frequently what attracts people to the nursing profession.

These life-affirming values, characteristic of being a nurse, are captured in the phrase "Nursing. It's real. It's life!" This was an advertising campaign launched in 2002 by Nurses for a Healthier Tomorrow[6] (*www.nursesource.org*), a coalition of national nursing and healthcare organizations whose mission is to heighten awareness about the nursing shortage and the opportunities available for those who seek a career in nursing.

Their 2007 campaign targets the shortage of nursing faculty and is called "Nursing Education … Pass It On." There has never been a more relevant time to be a nurse. Making a contribution to the world, making a difference in the lives of others, doing work that is more than just a job … that is what nurses do every day. It is the essence of nursing.

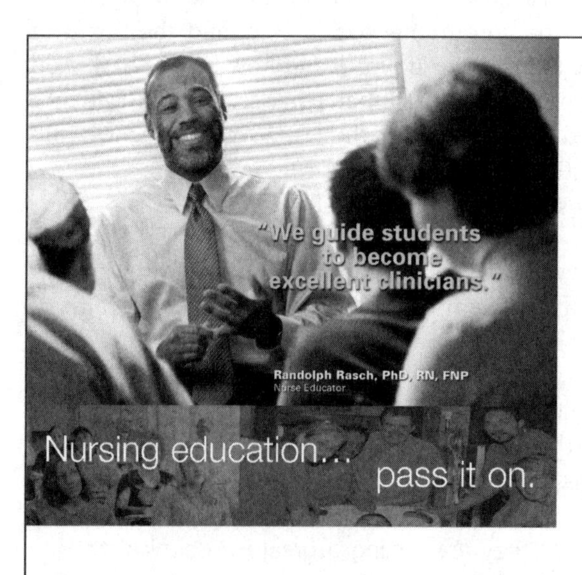

I teach my students to evaluate what they need to provide excellent patient care, access current knowledge so that care is cutting edge, and make a larger contribution to the health and welfare of the public. Mentoring is my passion. By sharing my story of nursing firsts, I am able to demonstrate how individuals from a variety of backgrounds can succeed. Want to learn more about the career advantages of nursing education? Visit us at: **www.nursesource.org**

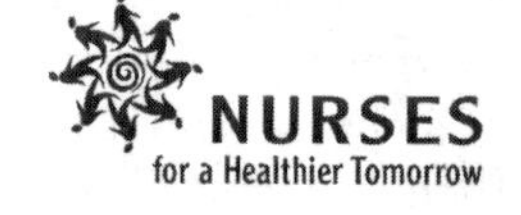

Nursing. It's Real. It's Life.

THE ESSENCE OF NURSING

To touch others and to be touched in return: this is what nursing is about. Nurses express and enact this life-affirming philosophy in many diverse ways every single day. And nurses often speak about getting as much as they give.

U.S. Army Captain Brian Gegel, a nurse anesthetist, felt his time in Iraq gave him a gift. He said, "You appreciate the freedoms our country offers, which are often taken for granted. You realize many day-to-day problems are not so important. I try to be a better person." (Reprinted with permission from *Report: The Official Newsletter of NYSNA* February 2005, Vol 35, No. 2).

Many nurses who served with relief organizations following the 2004 South Asian tsunami described their experiences as a source of personal growth. You can read about their experiences at *www.nurse.com*. Nurses were also front and center during the catastrophe that befell the nation's Gulf Coast in 2005 during Hurricane Katrina and its aftermath. They were seen refusing to abandon patients who could not be evacuated, caring for patients on life support who were being airlifted to safety, and obtaining leave from their jobs across the country to volunteer their services. For moving and inspiring personal accounts of these experiences, go to *nursingspectrum.com/katrina/*.

Jackie Cataldo, BSN, RN, is a nursing representative and organizer for the New York State Nurses Association, as well as an American Red Cross volunteer who serves on the Brooklyn Disaster Assistance Team. She wrote the poem that appears below, one of five of her reflections about September 11, 2001. While the smoke and debris to which Jackie refers was part of 9/11, it can also be seen as a metaphor for the experience many nurses have every day.

Other poems along with stories about the role of nurses on that day and thereafter, as well as scholarly articles written by nurses about responses to crises and disasters, can be found in the Spring/Summer 2002 issue of the *Journal of the New York State Nurses Association* (*http://nysna.org*).[8]

Smoke and Debris

Smoke and debris
Swirling mist in the artificial light.
Eeriness prevails the night.

Hell living through this tragedy.
Living?
Bodies mingled with concrete and steel.
Shattered glass and shreds of clothing.

Our mothers, fathers, sisters, brothers
and friends gone.
Breath crushed, seared from their lungs,
Hearts and children left alone. Pain.
Insurmountable pain for the buried
and the walking wounded.
Scream, I want to say to the rescue workers.
Eyes blank.
Staring at everything and nothing.
Scream your soul.

I want to touch your face,
Hold your mud-crusted hand.
You look into my eyes, holding tight
to my insides.
Your mouth almost smiles.
Energy low.
I smile for you.
Slowly, we pass each other and move
into the quiet thumping of the night.

In the June 3, 2002, issue of *Nursing Spectrum,* Janet Stevens,[9] the resource manager/clinical educator for the Nursing Education Department at Good Samaritan Hospital Medical Center in New York, wrote "Someone to Fill My Shoes," the story about how she found herself reflecting on what being a nurse meant when her daughter asked her, "What's the best part of being a nurse, Mommy?" What she said in this article reflects the essence of nursing.

> It [nursing] is an investment in my patients' lives. I make a difference every day—touching hearts and inspiring souls. This has been my passion for almost two decades. I am an ambassador of hope. I'm not famous and certainly not someone who brings home a six-digit yearly income. But the gifts of being a nurse are almost intangible. It's not measurable. Nursing has made me a better person, more patient, more understanding, and forgiving. I am in awe of the power of the human spirit. I appreciate the fragility of life and remind people to tell those who are precious to them how much they are loved. The World Trade Center's victims and their families gave us all this lesson. I'm reminded of this lesson every day. I am challenged to use leadership skills and motivated to connect with mentors and those they mentor. I nurture. I heal.... I get back so much more than I give. I am so blessed.

YOUR THREE-LEGGED STOOL OF CAREER SUCCESS

To succeed as a nurse means to take responsibility for and control the direction and the quality of your nursing practice by attending to three inextricably linked skill sets. You can envision these three skill sets as distinct but interrelated legs of a three-legged stool:

- Professional and clinical skills
- Career management skills
- Self-care skills and practice

Your nursing education, whether basic, graduate, or ongoing, comprises the professional/clinical leg of this three-legged stool.

Career seminars and resources, such as this book or online social networking groups, contribute to the career management leg.

Developing a self-care practice by learning to manage stress, attending personal development seminars, or seeking to enhance your self-awareness through psychotherapy are ways to ensure that the third leg has the same strength as the others. Chapter 15 will provide you with opportunities to explore further the development of self-care practice and what it can mean to your career and to the quality of your life as a whole.

Imagine what would happen if one or more of these legs were unevenly matched to the others. The stool would not be balanced. It would wobble and fail to support you. Neglecting one or more of the legs of this nursing practice trio is a prescription for stress, burnout, and compassion fatigue, and is likely to significantly hamper your ability to navigate the white water of change.

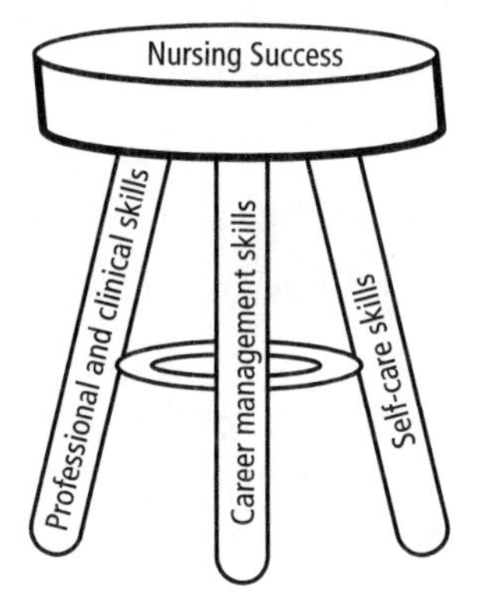

CHARACTERISTICS OF TODAY'S NURSE

The nurse who wants to have a successful career during these best and worst of times in healthcare without sacrificing personal well-being will learn to thrive on change, tracking the trends so as to be ready for what's new and what's next and committing to developing the characteristics below. As you read this list, use it to determine which characteristics you already have and which you need to develop. This list is not meant to be all-inclusive but, rather, an overview and introduction to the material you will find in the chapters that follow.

Nurses of today

- expect changes significant enough to alter their professional and personal lives at least every six months; they are adaptive and change-hardy.
- track emerging trends so that they are ready for what's new and what's next.
- can articulate the vision, mission, and values that drive their nursing practice.
- recognize the importance of having a BSN or are working toward it.
- participate in ongoing education in traditional as well as online venues.
- demonstrate leadership and are self-starters.
- are self-directed as well as team oriented.
- possess broad cross-training in nursing skills and competencies.
- seek certification from ANCC and/or other professionally recognized organizations.
- seek professional membership, including in the American Nurses Association and other associations or organizations relevant to their nursing practice specialties and interests.
- find mentors and are mentors to others.
- are technologically proficient, computer literate, and Internet savvy.
- are avid personal and professional networkers in traditional and online venues.
- consider themselves self-employed even as they work for others, realizing that while they are loyal to the job owned by their employer, they own their work.

- take their self-care practice as seriously as their professional/clinical skills, recognizing that one without the other neutralizes the effectiveness of both.
- utilize proactive behaviors and assertive communication styles.
- know their limits and are not afraid of using the word *no.*
- are flexible and creative thinkers.
- are willing to take informed risks and learn from their mistakes.
- never abdicate personal responsibility for themselves.

NURSES: THE PEOPLE IN THE PARENTHESES

We have become what psychologist and human potential expert Jean Houston, among others, calls "the people in the parentheses." These are the people suspended between what was and what will be. The healthcare industry and the nursing profession will continue to position and reposition themselves to meet the needs of patients and workers alike.

We belong to the generation of nurses bridging the gap between old and new, past and future, now and what will be. Life within these parentheses challenges our professional and personal wholeness and well-being as we work to maintain our footing in a constantly changing world. John Naisbitt, author of *Megatrends: Ten New Directions Transforming Our Lives,*[10] captures this well when he says:

> We are living in the time of the parentheses, the time between eras. Those who are willing to handle the ambiguity of this in-between period and to anticipate the new era will be a quantum leap ahead of those who hold on to the past. The time of the parentheses is a time of change and questioning. Although the time between eras is uncertain, it is a great and yeasty time, filled with opportunity. If we can learn to make uncertainty our friend, we can achieve much more than in stable eras. In stable eras, everything has a name and everything knows its place and we can leverage very little. But in the time of the parentheses we have extraordinary leverage and influence, individually, professionally, institutionally, if we can get a clear sense, a clear conception, and a clear vision, of the road ahead. My God, what a fantastic time to be alive!

And, what a fantastic time to be a nurse!

CHAPTER 2

Nursing Practice

> I make an earnest appeal to the nurses to remember the power and influence of their work and to improve it to the utmost.
>
> —*Susan B. Anthony, 1906*

Nursing is a knowledge-based profession; this significant fact is often neither fully understood nor appreciated. The nurse's ability to be a critical thinker and to use knowledge in the delivery of nursing care is essential to the well-being of those for whom nurses care. The basis for the scientific practice of nursing includes nursing science; the biomedical, physical, economic, behavioral, and social sciences; and ethics and philosophy. Nurses are concerned with human experiences and responses to birth, health, illness, and death. Nurses care for individuals, families, communities, and populations. In her book *Life Support: Three Nurses on the Front Lines*, Suzanne Gordon observes:

> Although nurses help us to live and die, in the public depiction of healthcare, patients seem to emerge from hospitals without ever having benefited from their assistance. Whether patients are treated in an emergency room in a few short hours, or on a critical care unit for months on end, we seem certain that physicians are responsible for all of the successes—or failures—in our medical system. In fact, we seem to believe that they are responsible not only for all of the curing, but for much of the caring. Nurses, on the other hand, remain shadowy figures moving mysteriously in the background.... In our high-tech medical system, nurses are the ones who care for the body and the soul... nurses are often closer to patients' needs and wishes than physicians... they spend far more time with patients and know them better.[1]

DEFINING NURSING PRACTICE

There are a variety of definitions of nursing practice. Florence Nightingale proposed that nursing practice involved being in "charge of the personal health of somebody... and what nursing has to do... is to put the patient in the best condition for nature to act upon him."[2] According to Virginia Henderson, nursing practice was "to assist the individual, sick or well, in the performance of those activities contributing to health or its recovery (or to a peaceful death) that he would perform unaided if he had the necessary strength, will, or knowledge, and to do this in such a way as to help him gain independence as rapidly as possible."[3] In many state nurse practice acts, the practice of professional nursing is defined as the diagnosis and treatment of human responses to actual or potential health problems. The American Nurses Association (ANA) proposes that there are seven essential features inherent in any definition of contemporary nursing practice:

1. Provision of a caring relationship that facilitates health and healing
2. Attention to the range of human experiences and responses to health, disease, and illness within the physical and social environments
3. Integration of assessment data with knowledge gained from an understanding and appreciation of the patient's or group's subjective experience
4. Application of scientific knowledge to the processes of diagnosis and treatment through the use of judgment and critical thinking
5. Advancement on professional nursing knowledge through scholarly inquiry
6. Influence on social and public policy to promote social justice
7. Assurance of safe, quality, and evidence-based practice[4]

THE LEGAL FOUNDATIONS OF NURSING PRACTICE

All registered professional nurses (RNs) are independent practitioners of the profession. Licensed practical nurses (LPNs) are dependent practitioners of nursing and deliver nursing care under the direction or supervision of an RN or otherwise authorized healthcare practitioner. The practice of nursing is authorized through state licensure. Nurses are held accountable to the laws, regulations, and rules of the state licensing authority and the standards and ethics of the profession as promulgated by the American Nurses Association and the specialty nursing organizations. It is a professional responsibility of a nurse to be a lifelong learner and to be knowledgeable of the legal and professional expectations associated with the practice of the profession. This includes applicable state laws and regulations governing nursing practice and the delivery of healthcare services.

In 2010, the American Nurses Association (ANA) published *Nursing's Social Policy Statement: The Essence of the Profession* in which the social contract that exists between nursing and society is expressed. In it is noted that "nursing's social contract reflects the profession's core values and ethics, which provide grounding for healthcare in society." The elements of nursing's social contract include the following:

- Humans manifest an essential unity of mind, body, and spirit.
- Human experience is contextually and culturally defined.
- Health and illness are human experiences. The presence of illness does not preclude health, nor does optimal health preclude illness.[5]
- The relationship between the nurse and patient occurs within the context of the values and beliefs of the patient and nurse.
- Public policy and the healthcare delivery system influence the health and well-being of society and professional nursing.
- Individual responsibility and interprofessional involvement are essential.[5]

In the United States, the legal authorization for nursing practice is contained in the Nurse Practice Acts of the states; in other nations, it is in the country's or province's applicable laws. Such acts can be general in the description of nursing practice or be very specific, listing authorized tasks or acts. Professional licensure has been established to protect the public from harm and to authorize the practice of a profession. States usually require a demonstration of attaining and successfully completing specific education, verification of minimal competency by passing the national nursing licensure examination (NCLEX-RN® exam), and evidence of good moral character. Licensure is a privilege, not a right. Once a nurse is authorized to practice the profession of nursing, the state expects that in all aspects of the nurse's life, there will be an awareness of this privilege and the nurse will remain personally committed to meeting any new educational requirements; maintaining appropriate competence in practice; and not engaging in any acts of professional misconduct, such as gross incompetence, negligence, fraud, conviction of a felony or misdemeanor, practicing while impaired, or specific unprofessional conduct acts as defined by the state (e.g., abusing a patient, failing to document one's practice appropriately, revealing personally identifiable information or facts about a patient, and inappropriately delegating professional acts).

In addition to the various state nurse practice acts, other state and federal laws can impact professional nursing practice. These include the conditions of participation of Medicare and Medicaid, the Emergency Medical Treatment and Active Labor Act (EMTALA), and various public health and/or state laws that mandate how healthcare facilities (hospitals, nursing homes, diagnostic and treatment centers, ambulatory/outpatient centers, home care agencies, hospices, assisted living facilities) must function in any specific jurisdiction. In addition, professional practice can be impacted by the availability or lack of reimbursement for nursing services from public and private insurers and by the credentialing requirements of such groups as the federal Departments of Education and Health and Human Services, the Centers for Medicare and Medicaid (CMS), The Joint Commission, and state or local health and education departments.

THE ETHICS OF NURSING

Nursing practice is based on an ethical tradition. ANA's *Code of Ethics for Nurses* explicitly expresses the primary goals, values, and obligations of the profession. The *Code* has two components—the nine provisions and the accompanying interpretative statements. The latter explain in greater detail each of the provisions and place the provision in the context of current nursing practice. The nine provisions are as follows:

1. The nurse, in all professional relationships, practices with compassion and respect for the inherent dignity, worth, and uniqueness of every individual, unrestricted by considerations of social or economic status, personal attributes, or the nature of health problems.
2. The nurse's primary commitment is to the patient, whether an individual, family, group, or community.
3. The nurse promotes, advocates for, and strives to protect the health, safety, and rights of the patient.
4. The nurse is responsible and accountable for individual nursing practice and determines appropriate delegation of tasks consistent with the nurse's obligation to provide optimum patient care.
5. The nurse owes the same duties to self as to others, including the responsibility to preserve integrity and safety, to maintain competence, and to continue personal and professional growth.
6. The nurse participates in establishing, maintaining, and improving healthcare environments and conditions of employment conducive to the provision of quality healthcare and consistent with the values of the profession through individual and collective action.

7. The nurse participates in the advancement of the profession through contributions to practice, education, administration, and knowledge development.
8. The nurse collaborates with other health professionals and the public in promoting community, national, and international efforts to meet health needs.
9. The profession of nursing, as represented by associations and their members, is responsible for articulating nursing values, for maintaining the integrity of the profession and its practice, and for shaping social policy.[6]

STANDARDS OF NURSING PRACTICE

ANA, in collaboration with the national specialty nursing organizations, has established standards of nursing practice for both generic and specialty nursing practice. The various standards describe a competent level of nursing care, reflect the values and priorities of the profession, provide direction for professional practice, and form a basis of accountability for all nurses regardless of practice setting. ANA's *Nursing: Scope and Standards of Practice* focuses on the processes of providing care (Standards of Care) and performing professional role activities (Standards of Professional Performance). The Standards of Practice describes a competent level of nursing care based on a critical-thinking model known as the nursing process and includes assessment, diagnosis, outcomes identification, planning, implementation, and evaluation. The Standards of Professional Performance describes a competent level of behavior in the professional nursing role and includes ethics, education, evidence-based practice, quality of practice, communication, leadership, collaboration, professional practice evaluation, resource utilization, and environmental health. Each standard consists of a standard statement (e.g., assessment—the registered nurse collects comprehensive data pertinent to the healthcare consumer's health and/or situation) and various identified competencies (e.g., elicits the healthcare consumer's values, preferences, expressed needs, and knowledge of the healthcare situation) for meeting the standard. These criteria are essential indicators of professional nursing practice, and all competencies must be met in order for the standard to be achieved.[7]

In addition, nurses can be held to local standards of nursing practice that describe what a reasonable and prudent nurse is expected to do. These local standards are usually the policies and procedures of the healthcare facility in which the nurse is employed. Employers' policies are considered essentially permission to practice nursing in that facility. These policies can limit the RN's legal scope of practice, but they cannot expand it. For instance, in most states, it is considered within the scope of practice of an RN to start an IV, but facilities do not have to let all RNs perform this procedure. The employer's policies and procedures must be in compliance with the state's Nurse Practice Act and any other laws, regulations, or rules that govern practice; they should reflect the professional standards of practice and address the expected ethical behavior.

NURSES' RIGHTS AND RESPONSIBILITIES

While the laws and regulations, standards of nursing practice, and the *Code of Ethics for Nurses* collectively address nurses' rights, obligations, and responsibilities, nurses sometimes feel puzzled regarding their rights and responsibilities. The New York State Nurses Association, in a paper discussing rights and responsibilities, defined a *right* as a just claim to something to which one is entitled, a prerogative, an entitlement, a political statement, or a legal declaration. In addition, a *responsibility* was defined as a trust or duty owed by one individual to another. The paper described three types of rights: fundamental human rights; legal rights, including those inherent in practice acts; and professional rights, such as the right to provide nursing care, the right to independent nursing practice judgment, the right to the necessary knowledge to safely practice, the right to ensure safe care environments, the right to advocate for the patient, the right to control the practice environment, the right to protest or refuse an unsafe practice assignment with the understanding of the risks and consequences involved, and the right to proper professional economic compensation. It is important to recognize that rights, regardless of the type, are not absolutes and choosing the "greater good" in professional practice involves risk taking and may have employment, legal, ethical, or disciplinary consequences.[8] According to ANA, the intrinsic linking of nurses' rights to professional responsibility can lead to frustration, a feeling of powerlessness, and a sense of inadequacy.[9] Dr. Claire Fagin, a distinguished nurse educator, has noted that nurses develop rights by having an image of themselves as being worthy of such rights, by sharing information about the profession and the work of nurses, by engaging in concerted advocacy, and by doing something for society that society values—not by being victims or pleading.[10] The New York State Nurses Association has observed that

> rights and responsibilities are segments of a single professional practice continuum. It is only through collective action that nurses can truly fulfill the responsibilities of nursing practice. As professional nurses, we will move forward learning the critical lessons of similar rights movements that strength and power are greater when pursued by a united group moving forward together.[11]

NURSING PRACTICE AND THE NURSING SHORTAGE

It is difficult to address nursing practice in this century without acknowledging the "elephant in the patient's room"—the national and global nursing shortage and its current and potential impact. In its materials, the ANA differentiates between a staffing shortage and a nursing shortage. A staffing shortage is a present-day concern and reflects "an insufficient number, mix, and/or experience of registered nurses and ancillary staff to safely care for the individual and aggregate needs of a specific patient population over a specific period of time." The nursing shortage is a more long-term concern and reflects "more of an economic perspective as the demand and need for registered nurses' services is greater than the supply of registered nurses who are qualified, available, and willing to work" (*Memo for CMA Executive Directors on Nursing's Agenda for the Future,* ANA 2002).[12]

Throughout the 20th century, there were cyclical periods identified as nursing shortages. Some of the quick fixes that were used to alleviate the various shortages included changes in work hours, financial bonuses for employment, increased wages, scholarships and grants to support education, attracting "second careerists" into the profession, foreign nurse recruitment, increased utilization of unlicensed assistive personnel, pay differentials and incentives for different shift work and specialty nursing, changes in practice modalities, and more attention to the contributions of the nursing staff by facilities and employers. However, the burdens associated with the work environment and the overall structure of the healthcare system in our nation were never adequately addressed.

The current nursing shortage is being impacted by the economics and financial issues of our times. When a nation experiences uncertain economic times, such as a recession, nurses, like other employees, are less likely to retire or leave the workforce. This quickly changes when the economic situation improves. However, the nursing workforce is continuing to age rapidly, and this factor alone will drive the shortage well into this century. Dr. Peter Buerhaus, a noted nurse workforce analyst, has projected that, despite the current easing of the shortage due to the recession, the U.S. nursing shortage will grow to 260,000 registered nurses by 2025.[13]

The good news is that the federal Bureau of Labor Statistics identifies nursing as one of the ten occupations projected to have the largest amount of openings in the next decade. There are 2.9 million nurses, making nursing the nation's largest healthcare profession.[14] By 2020, an article in the *Journal of Nursing Administration (JONA)* projects an estimated 400,000 RN vacancies with a lack of 650,000 baccalaureate-prepared nurses nationwide.[15] This shortage impacts all healthcare settings, not just hospitals. Finally, the economics of the country will impact these projections, as in difficult financial times, nurses are less likely to retire and more nurses tend to increase their work hours.

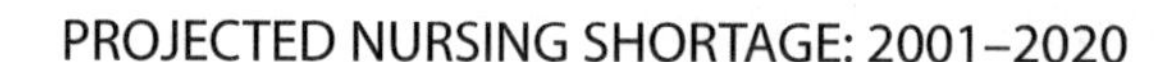

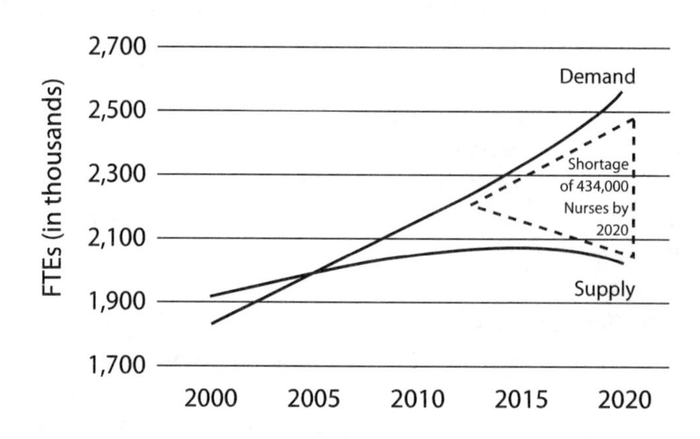

In April 2002, the Robert Wood Johnson Foundation (RWJ) released its report *Health Care's Human Crisis: The American Nursing Shortage*. Dr. Steven Schroder, RWJ president and CEO, comments:

> While we haven't seen a consumer backlash about the nursing crisis . . . there is more dissatisfaction out there than we are willing to acknowledge. . . . Consumers don't perceive the nursing shortage as an abstraction or a problem for hospital human resources departments to handle, but are already feeling its detrimental effect on the quality of care that they receive at the bedside. We must act soon.[16]

Of particular concern to the researchers is the fact that the nursing shortage endangers quality of care, places patients at risk, and could undermine the entire American healthcare industry. The report unequivocally states that the current nursing shortage will extend well into the 21st century and is driven by a broader and different set of factors than the shortages of the last century. These factors are identified as the following:

- The reality of an aging population, especially the 80 million baby boomers
- Fewer younger people entering the workforce, creating a "war for talent"
- The physical demands of nursing practice preventing most nurses from working past their mid-50s

- The lack of racial and ethnic diversity, especially of Hispanics, in the nursing workforce
- Women, as a result of the women's rights movement, choosing other professions over nursing and not enough men entering the profession to compensate for this change
- The perception by younger workers, such as those in Generation Y, that nursing is unappealing and does not address their needs and values
- Increased consumer activism
- A ballooning healthcare system with nurses lacking the authority to create and sustain change

The American Association of Colleges of Nursing (AACN) is particularly concerned about the struggle of universities and colleges to expand nursing enrollments to meet the increasing demand for nurses. In 2010, AACN launched the nation's first centralized application service for individuals looking to enroll in nursing education programs. This fully online system, known as NursingCAS, is available for students applying to RN programs offered at the baccalaureate, entry-level master's, associate degree, and diploma levels and to RNs applying to graduate nursing programs. The primary reason for this program is to ensure that the almost 55,000 seats left vacant each year in undergraduate and graduate nursing programs are filled, thus maximizing the educational capacity of the nation's schools of nursing (*www.nursingcas.org/About-NursingCAS.php*).

YOU AND YOUR NURSING PRACTICE

Control of your own nursing practice is essential. It is important for nurses to choose to work in environments that understand, value, and support each nurse's practice. As nursing practice evolves in the 21st century and the global nursing shortage is addressed, nurses need to assess carefully and systematically the complex dynamics that influence their ability to practice in any healthcare setting. This should begin with an honest and clear assessment of what is important to you as a nurse and what is essential in your practice. Be honest in your evaluation of your own skills and choose a practice setting that will take advantage of your skills, teach you new skills, increase your knowledge, and challenge you to grow. A state nurses association has suggested that information be obtained related to the following:

- The actual clinical practice that will be expected
- The availability of clinical preceptors on the direct care unit and master clinicians, such as clinical nurse specialists and nurse practitioners, to serve as resources and mentors

- Utilization of technical supports (computer systems, pharmacy dispersal, laboratory access)
- The availability of ancillary support (nursing assistants, housekeeping, dietary, transportation, clerical)
- Access to staff development and education
- Appropriate salaries and benefits
- Creative staffing and scheduling
- Contact with and responsiveness of nursing management.[17]

One way to find a supportive practice environment is to practice in a facility that has been granted Magnet Hospital status by the American Nurses Credentialing Center (ANCC). This program is based on a 1983 study by the American Academy of Nursing that sought to identify the characteristics of hospitals that were able to attract and retain professional nurses, even in times of shortage. The authors noted:

> The large number of instances in which the word "listen" is used by both the directors and the staff nurses .... Typical of the responses given by directors of nursing is this statement: "Listen to the staff... the best consultants are on your own staff." Staff nurses tend to say much the same thing ... listen to the patient contact people, they know what they are talking about."... It is the clear implication that the listening will be done well—that careful consideration is given to what is being said and the intent of utilizing the ideas set forth....[18]

The mission of the Magnet Recognition Program is to promote and recognize nursing excellence:

> Recognizing quality patient care, nursing excellence, and innovation in professional nursing practice, the Magnet Recognition Program provides consumers with the ultimate benchmark to measure the quality of care that they can expect to receive. When the *U.S. News & World Report* publishes its annual showcase of "America's Best Hospitals," being a Nurse Magnet facility contributes to the total score for quality of inpatient care. Of the 14 medical centers listed on the exclusive Honor Roll with the 2006 rankings (July 17, 2006) seven of the top ten were Magnet hospitals. (*www.nursingworld.org*)

Nurses should also seek facilities where evidenced-based practice (EBP) is supported and encouraged. Sigma Theta Tau (STT), the international nursing society, defines EBP as the integration of the best available evidence; nursing expertise; and the values and preferences of the patients, families, and communities served. EBP provides nurses with the opportunity to integrate current research and expert opinions on clinical practice into their own practice—direct care, administration, education, and research. Sigma Theta Tau collaborates with other nursing organizations in making available such resources as these:

- Nursing Knowledge International® (*www.nursingknowledge.org*) provides evidence-based knowledge solutions to help nurses help others.
- *Worldviews on Evidence-Based Nursing*™ is a peer-reviewed journal of knowledge synthesis and research on evidence-based practice.
- *Journal of Nursing Scholarship* is a quarterly journal containing peer-reviewed, thought-provoking articles from honor society members and leading nurse researchers.
- *ceLink*™ is the honor society's continuing education offering that includes more than 100 EBP case studies and articles.
- Virginia Henderson International Nursing Library (*www.nursinglibrary.org*) is an online, searchable resource of nursing research and conference abstracts.[19]

When choosing to work in facilities that use evidence-based practice, nurses should become involved in performance improvement projects that utilize research to tackle a clinical problem within their practice specialty. Dedication to this type of practice is essential to today's practitioners of nursing. Unfortunately, there is strong evidence that very few direct care nurses are involved in performance improvement initiatives, even with the Institute of Medicine identifying "evidence-based decision making" as Rule 5 in its *Ten Rules for Health Care*.[20] According to Melynk and Fineout-Overholt, without incorporating evidence-based practice into care, nursing practice becomes rapidly outdated and results in poor patient outcomes. Nurses who incorporate evidence-based practice into their care report higher levels of professional satisfaction and demonstrate more responsibility for their practice.[21]

DIRECTING YOUR PROFESSIONAL GROWTH

As discussed in other sections of this book, it is essential that all nurses have a clear direction for their own professional growth and use current and emerging information to know when changes need to be made in how and where they choose to practice nursing. This means making choices about educational and clinical advancement and specialty certification. Educational choices can include pursuing advanced degrees (master's or doctoral work) or continuing education courses. The most important educational goal for a registered nurse is to acquire a baccalaureate degree in nursing as early in one's career as possible. Nursing as a profession benefits from its multiple entry levels (diploma, associate degree, and baccalaureate degree); it suffers from not having enough nurses achieving the baccalaureate degree early in their careers. Without such a degree, nurses will encounter barriers to career mobility and advancement, and the profession will continue to have inadequate numbers of nurses with advanced degrees to teach and do research.

Clinical advancement can include deciding to become an advanced practice registered nurse (APRN), such as a nurse practitioner, clinical nurse specialist, nurse anesthetist, or nurse midwife, and/or deciding to specialize in a particular field of nursing. The designation APRN is recognized within the profession as a general term to describe the four nursing categories that require a master's degree or, increasingly, doctoral preparation. In some states, the title advanced practice registered nurse (APRN) or advanced practice nurse (APN) has been incorporated into the Nurse Practice Act as a legal designation. Additional descriptions of the practice of these nurses can be found in chapter 3.

Certification in a clinical (e.g., pediatrics, medical-surgical, psychiatric–mental health) or role (e.g., administrator, informatics, staff development) specialty is a way in which professional nurses demonstrate proficiency and expertise. Certification generally requires graduation from an accredited/approved educational program in the specialty, recommendations from professional colleagues, and satisfactory completion of a certification examination that is administered by the American Nurses Credentialing Center or a specialty nursing organization.

Staffing Issues

Significant research has linked safe nurse staffing and patient outcomes. Aiken found that the odds of patient mortality rose by 7 percent for every additional patient added to a nurse's assignment.[22, 23] It is quite clear that the nursing workplace environment must be enhanced to improve patient outcomes, reduce the burden on currently practicing nurses, provide an incentive for individuals to enter or return to nursing, and encourage nurses to stay active in the profession for longer periods. This includes the establishment of adequate and appropriate safe staffing.

Recently, there has been interest in legislatively mandating specific staffing ratios. The problem with this type of solution is that the established ratio, instead of being a minimum number, will more than likely become the maximum staffing level. Ratios also do not address differences among various healthcare facilities regarding patient acuity or encourage responding to shift-to-shift or unit-to-unit differences in staffing needs. It would be better to consider having the responsible health authority establish critical elements (e.g., patient acuity, census, skills of the staff, staff mix, geography of the unit, technology) that must be considered in any staffing methodology being used by a healthcare facility and let the facility, with input from its nurses, adapt the formula to its specific needs. The state could review the methodology for appropriateness and hold the facility responsible for meeting the established staffing levels.

Making Your Voice Heard

Many U.S. states (California, Florida, Illinois, Maine, Nevada, New Jersey, New York, Oregon, Rhode Island, Texas, Vermont, and Washington) and the District of Columbia have passed legislation and/or regulations that address nurse staffing. The states' activities range from requiring staffing studies, establishing safe staffing plans, and mandating the public reporting of nurse staffing levels to mandating specific nurse-to-patient ratios. In 1999, California was the first state to address staffing ratios by requiring the state's health department to establish specific nurse-to-patient ratios. The year before, Australia's province of Victoria established ratios but permitted nursing staff at the unit level to adjust the unit ratio to meet the specific needs of the patients. ANA has supported the federal Registered Nurse Safe Staffing Act, which would hold hospitals accountable for the development and implementation of valid nurse staffing plans. ANA has established a website dedicated to the issue of safe staffing, which provides nurses with the newest information on safe staffing, gives nurses access to safe staffing tools and resources, and provides nurses the opportunity to share their staffing stories and concerns. It can be accessed at *www.rnaction.org/site/PageServer?pagename=nstat_take_action_healthcare_reform*.

Mandatory and Voluntary Overtime

It is critical that employers stop relying upon mandatory overtime as a staffing method. In times of real emergencies or unexpected sick calls, many nurses voluntarily offer to work additional shifts. What today's nurses object to is the employer's reliance on routinely mandating overtime to staff a unit. This practice produces a tired, disgruntled, frustrated nurse who, in some circumstances, may be unsafe to continue to practice. After 16, 18, even 20 hours of work, how efficiently can any nurse be expected to deliver care in either a mandatory or voluntary overtime situation? Nurses also want to be able to meet their responsibilities to their families, including child and elder care. It is extremely unfortunate that some employers threaten nurses with charges of patient abandonment if they do not stay for the mandated overtime. Most states have very specific definitions of what legally constitutes patient abandonment. Nurses should be familiar with their state's rule on this issue and be prepared to protest formally any assignment that will create an unsafe practice situation for themselves and the patients.

Delegating

In today's healthcare environment, nurses are often asked to delegate or assign tasks to a variety of staff—other RNs, LPNs or nursing assistive personnel (NAPS, formerly referred to as unlicensed assistive personnel or UAPS). The differences and distinctions between delegating and assigning differ from state to state. Therefore, all nurses should make sure that they understand what is legally permitted in their states of licensure. Generally, it is illegal for a registered nurse to permit another RN, LPN, or NAP to perform any task that the RN knows the staff member is not qualified to perform by reason of licensure, education, or competency. Nurses must develop a clear understanding of what constitutes the protected scope of nursing practice and use this understanding to make appropriate assignments and to ensure that the public receives safe and effective nursing care. Therefore, it is important that RNs know the competencies of other RNs, the competencies and legal practice of LPNs, and the types of tasks that can be performed by a NAP.

The American Association of Critical Care Nurses (AACN) has developed a list of six risk factors that an RN could use when evaluating if assistive personnel should perform a certain task on a particular patient. These risk factors are potential for harm, condition/stability of the patient, complexity of the task, the level of problem solving or innovation that might be needed, the unpredictability of the outcome, and the level of interaction required with the patient to complete the task successfully. An expected professional standard is that the RN will provide the appropriate level of direction and supervision when any nursing care is being delivered by assistive personnel.[24]

Malpractice

Nurses are increasingly concerned that the staffing problems in the workplace will result in disciplinary actions, criminal charges, or civil malpractice suits. Malpractice is the type of negligence that occurs when a professional violates a standard of care of the profession. Nursing malpractice occurs when a nurse makes a mistake that harms a patient and the mistake is one that a reasonably careful and competent nurse would not have made in a similar situation. Insurance carriers have identified some practice categories that can lead to malpractice litigation:

- Nonadherence to basic or fundamental nursing protocol (e.g., administering an unknown medication)
- Failure to recognize signs and symptoms of a medical condition or complications (e.g., inadequate assessment)
- Failure to intervene appropriately (e.g., failure to report changes in a patient's condition)
- Improper performance of psychomotor skills (e.g., nonadherence to principles of asepsis)
- Failure to act as a patient advocate and ensure that competent treatment was received (e.g., acceptance of a passive "do what you are told" role)
- Inadequate communication between the nurse and the patient, nursing supervisor, and/or physician (e.g., failure to listen to and convey an understanding of the patient's complaints and needs)
- Failure to adhere to the nurse's role as a teacher (e.g., lack of teaching about medication management and drug side effects)

To decrease the incidence of malpractice charges, it is essential for nurses to assess the patient on a regular basis and report changes as needed to the MD, NP, PA, and/or nursing supervisor, remembering to document and communicate clearly with the patient and the family. It is also prudent for nurses to have their own malpractice insurance. Often nurses rely on the employer's insurance. However, this insurance covers only incidents that occur when one is actually working. Since one is always legally a nurse, any advice or care that is rendered outside of the employment situation can result in malpractice claims. While most states have Good Samaritan laws, one would still have to prove that the law applied to the situation being litigated. Malpractice insurance should provide coverage for each claim and aggregate claims, a defendant expense benefit, a personal injury liability, deposition representation, and defense of disciplinary charges.

POLITICAL ACTIVISM

Increasingly, nurses are engaging in grassroots legislative activities and political action to promote nursing's agenda for healthcare; to improve workplace conditions; and to provide funding for nursing scholarships, grants, and research. ANA has successfully lobbied Congress for the passage of laws providing monies to boost nursing school enrollments, encourage nurses to return to school for advanced degrees, and support the utilization of the Magnet Hospital criteria in healthcare facilities. ANA was particularly disappointed when the Department of Labor rescinded the Ergonomics Program Standards after the ANA had worked two years for its passage. Nurses, as they age, are increasingly concerned about the lack of adequate ergonomic guidelines and rules, especially with the number of work-related musculoskeletal injuries they experience. While ANA continues to work with Congress to achieve passage of comprehensive ergonomics legislation that applies to all healthcare settings, it has its own successful campaign called Handle With Care. Its aim is to prevent back and musculoskeletal injuries through education and training and the increased use of assistive equipment and patient-lifting devices.

ANA supported the Obama administration's healthcare reform initiatives and passage of the *Affordable Care Act* (2010), noting that it clearly represents a movement toward much-needed comprehensive and meaningful reform for our nation's healthcare system. RNs are fundamental to the critical shift needed in health services delivery, with the goal of transforming the current "sick care" system into a *true* "healthcare" system. ANA noted that the new system incorporates primary, preventative, transitional, and home care into the current acute care–focused, hospital-based health system in the United States. Other issues being addressed on a federal level by ANA in collaboration with other nursing organizations include the following: maintaining access to Medicare and Medicaid, safe staffing, violence against healthcare workers, toxic chemicals, safe patient handling, and APRN practice. Nursing has a long tradition of addressing social and political issues that affect our patients and communities—it is a hallmark of the profession dating back to Florence Nightingale.

Political action committees (PACs) are one way that individuals and groups can gain access to legislators and other elected officials. PACs endorse and support candidates and officeholders. Through grassroots activities, nursing PACs encourage nurses to contact politicians, specifically their own representatives, and get nursing's message out. This message can be heard through financial support, campaign assistance, and voting. The democratic process requires the involvement of all citizens, and getting nursing's message out requires that nurses learn to share their knowledge and experiences with candidates, legislators, and officeholders. The largest nursing PAC is the American Nurses Association's, which can be accessed at *nursingworld.org/MainMenuCategories/ANAPoliticalPower/ANAPAC.aspx*.

CHANGING THE FUTURE OF NURSING

Both the staffing and nursing shortages have produced a unique opportunity for nurses, the nursing profession, and all other interested stakeholders to stop the cyclical nursing shortages once and for all. But one can question whether or not the stakeholders are motivated to change this cycle. The healthcare industry has failed to appreciate that in many healthcare settings, the main commodity provided is nursing care, not medical care. This is not said to diminish the value of the services provided by our physician colleagues but to emphasize that often, most of the care required by patients in hospitals, nursing homes, clinics, home care, and hospices is nursing care. Unfortunately, the healthcare industry, in its convoluted struggles with managed care, cost cutting, changes in reimbursement, onerous regulations, increasing demands of technology, and burdensome documentation, has not been able to construct a workplace environment that supports the delivery of nursing care to the satisfaction of both the nurses and the patients. It is also reluctant to provide adequate compensation for nursing care. The workplace environment, including improved communication between direct care nurses and nursing management and administration, staffing flexibility and appropriate staffing formulas, no mandatory overtime, adequate compensation, minimization of hazards, and promotion of safety, must be addressed to support both retention and recruitment. It is essential to establish a strong base of nurses within the profession who have baccalaureate degrees to ensure that the knowledge needed for increasingly complex nursing care is supported. Also needed are increased technological support, reduction of unnecessary and redundant paperwork, recruitment of more men and minorities, and improvement of the media's and public's image of nursing.

The nation has for decades struggled with how to develop from the complex healthcare industry a true and functional healthcare system for all that would ensure access to safe, quality, affordable services.

ANA's *Health System Reform Agenda* calls for a fundamental reform of the current healthcare system to create one that is responsive to the needs of patients and provides equal access to safe, quality care for every citizen and resident in a cost-effective manner. In the *Agenda*, ANA supports the following:

- Healthcare is a basic human right. The current healthcare system needs to be restructured to ensure universal access to a standard package of essential healthcare services for all citizens and residents.
- The development and implementation of health policies should reflect the Institute of Medicine's six aims—safe, effective,

patient-centered, timely, efficient, and equitable and should be based on outcomes research that ultimately saves money for the system.

- The system must be reshaped and redirected away from an overuse of expensive, technology-driven, hospital-based acute care services toward a balance between high-tech treatment and community-based and preventive services with a focus on primary care.
- The most desirable option for financing a reformed healthcare system is a single-payer mechanism.

It is imperative that nurses and the profession be involved in charting the future of healthcare in our nation, as the future of healthcare is intrinsically linked to the future of the nursing profession.

KNOWLEDGE AND INSPIRED CARING

Nursing and nurses are essential to the delivery of healthcare in this nation. The fact that the profession remains often misunderstood should not be viewed as a negative but as an inspiration. Nurses need to be inspired to proclaim nursing's work and identify the beneficial outcomes of our practice. Nurses must be inspired to understand the full scope of nursing practice and to protect it from being diminished. We need to be inspired to accept full responsibility for our own personal, lifelong learning and to plan our careers. The career path that will support our practice of the profession of nursing deserves to be inspirationally planned, not allowed merely to occur haphazardly. Nurses need to be inspired to remember that the focus of nursing practice is the patient, whether an individual, family, community, or population. Nursing practice is knowledge combined with inspired caring; it will forever remain both an art and a science.

CHAPTER 3

Nursing Education

> It has always seemed strange to me that in our endless discussions about education so little stress is laid on the pleasure of becoming an educated person, the enormous interest it adds to life. To be able to be caught up into the world of thought—that is to be educated.
>
> —*Edith Hamilton*

The professional nursing role of the present and future calls for nurses to practice within a complex healthcare system, to work as peers in interdisciplinary teams, and to be able to integrate evidence-based clinical knowledge with knowledge of diverse communities and their resources. As healthcare delivery grows increasingly complex, so does the nurse's scope of practice, requiring ongoing clinical and educational preparation for new challenges and increasing expectations. In this environment, nurses must possess a broad perspective and understanding of health and factors affecting health and be able to utilize critical thinking, problem-solving, and communication skills effectively. Not only is advanced and continuing nursing education required to meet these challenges, but it is essential for quality patient care, for the advancement of the profession, and for your actualization as a nurse. The nursing profession subscribes to a philosophy of lifelong learning, which allows you to prepare yourself for a multitude of nursing roles and innovative opportunities. Nurses prepared at all educational levels have important roles to play in this evolving healthcare system.

The material in this chapter will assist you in directing your professional growth and is designed to give you the information you need to make informed choices about your nursing education, including basic entry-level programs, master's level programs, and doctoral programs, as well as options for advanced practice, professional certification, and continuing education. Refer to the print and online resources at the back of this book for still more information.

YOUR BELIEFS ABOUT NURSING EDUCATION

Place a check mark next to the statement below that is closest to your belief about nursing education:

- ❐ I know it's important to keep learning, but honestly, how can I fit it into my schedule? I'm exhausted from my life as it is; how can I think of adding school on top of everything else I'm doing? I'm working full-time and about to have my third child, and my parents need my attention more these days.
- ❐ I enjoy learning. There's no way to be an effective nurse today without a solid education to begin with and ongoing learning to keep current. But it's hard to figure out how to do it. I was attending in-service education programs at my hospital until a few months ago when staffing got worse and made it too difficult. So I've begun to explore the online CE sites, and I'm talking to other nurses on my listserv to hear what they are doing.
- ❐ I did my stint in school. It didn't teach me the skills I needed to be a nurse. I learned that from my preceptor. There's no way I'm wasting my time on something like that again. I'm just glad it's over. If this hospital wants me to get more education, let them pay for it and give me the time off to do it. Otherwise, forget it!

Most likely, your response was some combination of the first two sets of comments. You know that education is important and are committed to it, but you might have difficulty juggling it along with your other responsibilities. If your belief about nursing education is reflected in the third response, you are marching out of step with present-day thinking as well as the professional nursing community and are likely to find yourself with relatively limited career options and opportunities.

ESSENTIAL TRUTHS ABOUT EDUCATION

A few ideas about education seem important to state. Ask yourself how closely you agree with the following facts:

- ❐ Education is a process, not an end point. Things change. The faster they change, the more there is to learn.
- ❐ The goal of education is to teach you how to learn about what you need to know, giving you the latest example of how this looks and where you might be using it.
- ❐ It is up to you to ensure that you continue learning when the "next new thing" arrives, whether it is technology, a different procedure,

or another conceptual framework within which to operate, such as evidence-based practice.

- ❒ Whether or not your employer provides you with incentives to learn, financial or otherwise, it is still essential to ensure that ongoing nursing education remains one of your professional priorities, especially since it is a standard of nursing practice and often required for license renewal or certification.
- ❒ Your commitment to nursing education and clinical advancement provides a clear direction for your professional growth, including how and where you will be able to practice nursing.

THE NURSING SHORTAGE: THE NEED TO RECRUIT AND EDUCATE MORE NURSES

As discussed in chapters 1 and 2, the United States will continue to have a shortage of nurses for quite some time. By 2020, the national shortage is projected to increase to more than 1 million full-time equivalent (FTE) nursing positions (Figure 3.1) if current trends continue, suggesting that only 64 percent of projected demand will be met (Figure 3.2; see *bhpr.hrsa.gov/healthworkforce/reports/nursing/rnbehindprojections/4.htm#x24*). Keep in mind that the state of the American economy and the efforts of healthcare employers to retain mature nurses are potential mitigating factors to this gloomy forecast. Nurses may stay in the workforce, or those who have left may return. Refer to chapters 1, 2, 6, and 7 for broader discussions of this topic.

It is clear that the recruitment and education of nurses has become an urgently important priority for the nursing profession. You may want to avail yourself of the following means to address this potential crisis and opportunities:

- Schools and colleges of nursing are amplifying their efforts to recruit eligible students by expanding their programs and increasing the flexibility of class schedules to meet the needs of busy adults. Watch for innovative programs and the increased availability of distance-learning programs, which allow you to take courses online.
- Special recruitment campaigns are being developed to recruit men and minority students, both of which are underrepresented populations in the nursing profession. You can track programs of interest though the ANA (*nursingworld.org*) and the American Association of Colleges of Nursing (AACN; *www.aacn.nche.edu*).

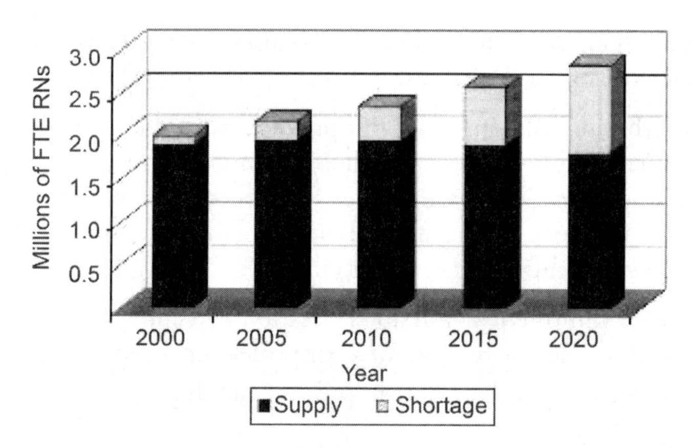

Figure 3.1 Projected U.S. FTE RN Shortages, 2000 to 2020

Another resource is the website of the journal *Minority Nurse* (*minoritynurse.com*). Also, refer to chapters 1 and 7 for discussions of the innovative recruitment campaigns called "The Campaign for Nursing's Future" and "Nursing, It's real. It's life!"

- Consider taking advantage of the increased availability of financial assistance and loan forgiveness programs if you are ready to advance or continue your education. One example is the 2002 Nurse Reinvestment Act. This bill authorizes increased loans for nursing students and for nurses seeking advanced degrees. Two of the many nursing websites that will track the progress of this funding, including its availability, the dollar amount allotted, and the stipulations for eligibility, are the American Nurses Association (*nursingworld.org*) and the American Association of Colleges of Nursing (*aacn.nche.org*).

	2000	**2005**	**2010**	**2015**	**2020**
Supply	1,890,700	1,942,500	1,941,200	1,886,100	1,808,000
Demand	2,001,500	2,161,300	2,347,000	2,569,800	2,824,900
Shortage	(110,800)	(218,800)	(405,800)	(683,700)	(1,016,900)
Supply ÷ Demand	94%	90%	83%	73%	64%
Demand Shortfall	6%	10%	17%	27%	36%

Figure 3.2 Projected U.S. FTE RN Supply, Demand, and Shortages

- Watch for healthcare organizations to offer incentives for nursing education, especially for advanced practice roles, which are anticipated to be in short supply as the need for primary care increases.

THE FACULTY SHORTAGE: THE NEED TO RECRUIT AND EDUCATE MORE FACULTY

The statistics about the shortage of nursing faculty and its effect on educating qualified nurses are cause for great concern. U.S. nursing schools turned away over 40,000 qualified applicants from baccalaureate and graduate nursing programs in 2007 due to an insufficient quantity of faculty, clinical sites, classroom space, and clinical preceptors and budget constraints (AACN 2007–08). In 2006, a total of 42,866 students were turned away from these nursing programs as well. Almost three quarters of the nursing schools responding to a 2007 AACN survey pointed to faculty shortages as a reason for not accepting all qualified applicants into entry-level baccalaureate programs (*www.aacn.nche.edu/IDS/*).

According to AACN, the average ages of doctorally prepared nursing faculty holding the ranks of professor, associate professor, and assistant professor were 59.1, 56.1, and 51.7 years, respectively. For master's-prepared nursing faculty, the average ages for professors, associate professors, and assistant professors were 58.9, 55.2, and 50.1 years, respectively (*www.aacn.nche.edu/IDS/*).

Since many nurses delay getting advanced degrees, which would enable them to teach at the collegiate level, and some do not even consider nursing education as a career choice until they are older, the number of years that the nurse educator will spend teaching may be limited. In 2002, the average age of nurse faculty at retirement was 62.5 years, and a wave of retirements is expected within the next ten years (*Nursing Outlook* 2002). In fact, it is projected that between 200 and 300 faculty prepared at the doctoral level will be eligible for retirement each year through 2012, and between 220 and 280 master's-prepared nurse faculty will be eligible for retirement between 2012 and 2018 (*www.us.elsevierhealth.com/product.jsp?isbn=00296554*).

Strategies, including legislation to address the faculty shortage, are discussed below. Many opportunities exist among these strategies for those interested in nursing education as a career choice.

- There is aggressive marketing within the nursing community and to the public along with the development of financial incentives and scholarships, including the support of federal funding such as the 2002 Nurse Reinvestment Act. Creative strategies are also being tested to allow senior nurse faculty members to continue working with reduced schedules. For a broader discussion of workplace accommodations designed to make it easier for mature nurses, including nursing faculty, to remain in the workforce, refer to chapter 6. You can also access *www.aacn.nche.edu* for the most recent policy and governmental actions to support education for nurses.

- Senator Richard Durbin (D-IL) introduced the Troops to Nurse Teachers Act of 2008 (TNT), which would permit active duty and retired Nurse Corps Officers to serve as faculty in schools of nursing. Modeled after the Department of Defense's Troops to Teachers program, TNT would create a fellowship program for commissioned officers with a graduate nursing degree, a scholarship program for commissioned officers who have served at least 20 years of active duty as nurses, a transitional assistance program for Nurse Corps officers who have served at least 20 years and are already qualified to teach, and a program for retired Nurse Corps officers who can serve as full-time faculty in a accredited school of nursing (*www.aacn.nche.edu/media/newsreleases/2008/tntact.html*).
- AACN and Johnson & Johnson's "Campaign for Nursing's Future" announced the first scholarship recipients for the newly created Minority Nurse Faculty Scholars program. Created to address the nation's shortage of nurse educators and the need to diversify the faculty population, this program provides financial support to graduate nursing students from minority backgrounds who agree to teach in a school of nursing after graduation (*www.aacn.nche.edu/media/newsreleases/2008/j&jscholars.htm*).
- AACN's annual inaugural Faculty Development Conference in 2008 was aimed at helping nurses transition to faculty roles in baccalaureate and higher degree programs. More than 250 new and future nursing faculty attended this event titled "Transforming Learning, Transforming People." The program is now offered annually (*www.aacn.nche.edu/conferences/08facdev.htm*).
- Many statewide initiatives are underway to address both the shortage of registered nurses and nurse educators. In October 2006, AACN released an Issue Bulletin titled "State Legislative Initiatives to Address the Nursing Shortage" describing dozens of these efforts, including comprehensive programs in Maryland, Kansas, Colorado, Illinois, and Utah. Specific strategies that address the faculty shortage include loan forgiveness programs, faculty fellowships, and salary

supplements can be found at *www.aacn.nche.edu/publications/issues/Oct06.htm* and *www.aacn.nche.edu/government/stateresources.htm.*

- Representatives Nita Lowey (D-NY), Peter King (R-NY), and Lois Capps (D-CA) introduced the Nurse Education, Expansion and Development Act (NEED) in the House, and a companion bill was introduced in the Senate by Senator Richard Durbin (D-IL). The NEED Act would amend Title VIII of the Public Health Service Act to authorize capitation grants (formula grants) for nursing schools to increase the number of faculty and students. Capitation grant programs have been used effectively to address past nursing shortages (*www.aacn.nche.edu/government/pdf/capgrants.pdf*).
- AACN and the California Endowment launched a scholarship and mentorship program in 2006 to increase the number of minority nursing faculty in California. Through this program, nursing students from underrepresented backgrounds are eligible to receive up to $18,000 in funding support to complete a graduate nursing degree. In exchange, students engage in leadership development activities and commit to teaching in a California nursing school after graduation (*www.aacn.nche.edu/CAEAwardApp.pdf*).
- The U.S. Secretary of Education designated nursing as an "area of national need" for the first time under the Graduate Assistance in Areas of National Need (GAANN) program. As a result of this AACN-led lobbying effort, a new funding stream for PhD programs in nursing was created. In April 2006, $2.4 million in grant funding through the GAANN programs was awarded to 14 schools of nursing (*www.ed.gov/programs/gaann/index.html*).

This is an opportune time for nurses interested in academic careers. Stay alert for recruitment incentives, such as federally funded master's and doctoral programs, to be more available. See Resources at the end of the book to learn more.

LEVELS OF NURSING EDUCATION

The American Association of Colleges of Nursing specifies three levels of education for the preparation of professional nurses. These are the baccalaureate, master's, and doctoral degrees. Although the baccalaureate is the primary pathway to professional nursing practice and is preferred by healthcare employers and offers the greatest career mobility for the nurse, there are three other entryways: the two-year associate's degree in nursing, the three-year hospital diploma, and the accelerated bachelor of science in nursing (BSN) or generic master's programs for those who have degrees in fields other than nursing.

In keeping with long-term trends, 59 percent of all new graduates eligible to enter the nursing workforce this year in the United States were prepared in two-year associate degree programs, 38 percent graduated from baccalaureate nursing programs, and 8 percent graduated from diploma programs (*www.prweb.com/releases/2008/03/prweb734894.htm*).

The Bachelor's Degree in Nursing

The Bachelor of Science Degree in Nursing (BSN) typically takes four years and provides a liberal arts education in the sciences and humanities along with preparation for nursing. The BSN curriculum includes a strong focus on the development of intellectual skills, as well as scientific, critical thinking, humanistic, communication, and leadership skills. Courses in community health and nursing research are also requirements of baccalaureate education. While technical skills are essential to nursing practice, baccalaureate education emphasizes the additional importance of the critical thinking and problem-solving skills, which establish the basis for using clinical judgment essential for working in today's evidence-based healthcare settings. Baccalaureate nursing programs are far more likely than other entry-level programs to provide students with on-site clinical experiences in settings outside the hospital. As a result, the BSN graduate is well prepared for practice in such sites as home health agencies, outpatient centers, and neighborhood clinics, where opportunities are expanding as hospitals focus more on acute care and health services move beyond the hospital to primary and preventive care sites throughout the community. Baccalaureate education, with its broader, more scientific base, provides the soundest foundation for the wide variety of nursing roles and is required for entry into advanced nursing practice and education. Despite this fact, only 43.6 percent of the nursing workforce holds a baccalaureate degree (*bhpr.hrsa.gov/nursing/NACNEP/reports/first/3.htm*).

ANCC Magnet-accredited hospitals prefer baccalaureate-prepared nurses wherever possible, as studies show that hospitals utilizing nurses with BSNs have lower patient morbidity and mortality rates. A landmark study conducted by Dr. Linda Aiken, a nurse educator and researcher, found that surgical patients have a "substantial survival advantage" if treated in hospitals with higher proportions of nurses educated at the baccalaureate or higher degree level. A 10 percent increase in the proportion of nurses holding BSN degrees decreased the risk of patient death and failure-to-rescue by 5 percent. The authors of this study recommend that public financing of nursing education be directed at shaping a workforce best prepared to meet the needs of the population. They also call for renewed support and incentives from nurse employers to encourage registered nurses to pursue education at the baccalaureate and higher degree levels (*www.aacn.nche.edu/media/factsheets/ImpactEdNP.htm*).

In February 2007, the Council on Physician and Nurse Supply released a statement calling for a national effort to expand baccalaureate nursing programs substantially. The Council noted that a growing body of research supports the relationship between the level of nursing education and both the quality and safety of patient care. Consequently, the group is calling on policymakers to shift federal funding priorities in favor of supporting more baccalaureate-level nursing programs (*www.aacn.nche.edu/media/factsheets/ImpactEdNP.htm*).

The Accelerated BSN Program

For students who have a baccalaureate degree in another field, this accelerated BSN option could be an excellent choice, particularly for people interested in nursing as a second career. Typically, students attend classes full-time and earn a BSN in as little as 12 months, assuming all science and other prerequisites have been satisfied. Programs may vary in length between 12 and 18 months. The curriculum contains the same courses and clinical hour requirements as the traditional BSN program but is more compact and, as a result, more rigorous, as well as intellectually and physically demanding. Additional information about these programs, including a comprehensive list of accelerated baccalaureate programs, is in the April 2008 AACN *Issue Bulletin* entitled "Accelerated Programs: The Fast-Track to Careers in Nursing" at *www.aacn.nche.edu/publications/issues/Aug02.htm.*

The Associate Degree in Nursing

Obtaining an Associate's Degree in Nursing (ADN) typically takes two years. The program is offered at community colleges or at hospital-based schools of nursing. You may also see this educational credential referred to as Associate in Applied Science (AAS). The two years of education are devoted to the development of nursing skills and competencies. These nurses are adept at providing direct patient care in acute care or long-term care settings.

Many nurses prepared at this level go on to obtain the BSN degree. New York State has legislation pending to require the ADN graduate to earn a BSN within ten years of obtaining first licensure. Many employers offer nurses tuition reimbursement to assist them with returning to school while they work.

The ADN as an Entryway, Not an End

The ADN is a faster and less expensive entryway into professional nursing practice than the BSN degree, but it has limitations. You would be wise to weigh carefully the result of allowing this to remain your terminal degree, meaning the only formal preparation you have to offer a healthcare employer. Be clear about the potential limitations of the associate's degree and commit yourself to adding the BSN credential, either through the articulation programs described below or after working for a period of time as a direct care nurse and then returning to school. Nurses who choose this method of nursing education can often benefit from tuition reimbursement offered by their employers if they return to school part-time and continue working.

Articulation Programs

These are sometimes called "degree-completion" programs, in which a signed agreement between a baccalaureate program and an associate degree program provide a kind of seamless pipeline for the ADN graduate to obtain the BSN degree. The collaborative efforts of and agreements between a particular ADN and BSN program permit the advancement of the ADN student's education in the most facilitative way possible. Because of the predetermined, collaborative efforts of both educational institutions, students are ensured the best use of both programs. The result is a win-win outcome for the student as well as for the educational programs, in that time and money are utilized most efficiently and credits are not needlessly lost. Articulation agreements can vary greatly.

The Master's Degree in Nursing

The nurse who desires clinical, academic, research, policy, or administrative advancement will need a master's degree and possibly a doctoral degree as well. Admission to graduate nursing programs requires a baccalaureate degree and the achievement of acceptable scores on such entry exams as the Graduate Record Exam (GRE) and/or the Miller Analogies Test. These programs are about two years in length and typically include a research component in the form of a thesis or comprehensive graduate-level project.

The master's-prepared nurse functions in advanced practice roles, including health promotion, the management and delivery of primary healthcare, and case management of the acutely or chronically ill patient. This nurse is also prepared for roles in community health, research, policy formulation, education, and administration. Nurses prepared at the master's level are qualified to become managers and administrators of healthcare organizations, including the directors of divisions and departments of nursing and nursing services. Increasingly, the doctoral degree is preferred for administrators and nurse executives, along with the Master of Business Administration (MBA). Many nurse administrators/executives add the MBA to their master's and doctoral preparation in nursing. Master's-prepared nurses are also qualified to teach in colleges and schools of nursing, although they are often limited to adjunct faculty or clinical teaching roles in baccalaureate programs. They may be full-time faculty in ADN programs. For nurses seeking full-time, tenure-track academic appointments in a university setting, the doctoral degree is necessary. There is a tremendous lack of RNs for qualified faculty positions. Nursing education programs at all levels, from practical nursing education to doctoral nursing education, employed 46,655 RNs in March 2000.

The master's degree also prepares the advanced practice registered nurse (APRN), which is the global term used for the following specializations: the nurse practitioner (NP), the clinical nurse specialist (CNS), the certified registered nurse anesthetist, (CRNA), and the certified nurse midwife (CNM). These roles are described below. Credentials for master's degrees vary by state and include MS or MSN as a first professional degree in nursing or a master of science (MS) with a nursing major, such as psychiatric/mental health. Examples include the following:

- **MSN:** Master of Science in Nursing with a specialty in nursing
- **MNSc:** Master in Nursing Science
- **MEd:** Master in Education with a major in nursing
- **MA:** Master of Arts with a major in nursing

Nurse Practitioner (NP)

Nurse practitioners may provide all primary care services, including full history and physicals, the administration of immunization protocols, the ordering and interpretation of X-rays and laboratory data, and the prescription of medications. They practice in a variety of specialties, such as adult health, pediatrics, women's health, family health, as well as psychiatry and mental health. They can prescribe medications in all states, with 18 states authorizing this practice as an independent function without requiring physician collaboration. They work in clinics and hospitals in metropolitan and rural areas, especially in places with underserved healthcare needs, and in private practice. Professional certification is usually required by employers and insurance companies that provide reimbursement of healthcare expenses. The NP has more broadly defined functions than the clinical nurse specialist (CNS).

Clinical Nurse Specialist (CNS)

This nurse has highly specialized skills and is prepared to practice in a wide variety of healthcare settings, including psychiatric/mental health, community health, oncology, pediatrics, and so on. Primary roles in which the CNS functions often include acting as a patient advocate, as well as educator, clinical resource, consultant, and role model to other nurses, especially those practicing at the generalist level. The clinical nurse specialist can be found in all employment sectors of the healthcare industry as well as in private practice. The psychiatric clinical nurse specialist often has an independent psychotherapy practice and, unlike those in other CNS specialties, is considered a primary care provider. Just like the NP, professional certification as a CNS is typically required or, at the very least, advantageous.

Certified Registered Nurse Anesthetist (CRNA)

This master's-prepared nurse graduates from a certified nurse anesthesia program and administers anesthetic agents, provides pre- and postanesthesia care, performs emergency resuscitation, and provides acute and chronic pain management. Employment settings include hospitals, surgicenters, emergency rooms, and physician's offices. Professional certification is required.

Certified Nurse Midwife (CNM)

This nurse graduates from an accredited nurse midwifery program and provides prenatal care, labor and delivery care, neonatal care, family planning, and well-woman care. The CNM has a formal, collaborative relationship with an obstetrician, who provides consultation as well as management of high-risk patients. CNMs are employed in hospitals, freestanding clinics and birth centers, ambulatory sites, and physician's offices. Professional certification is required.

The Generic Master's Degree in Nursing

The generic master's program is for those who are not yet nurses and have a baccalaureate or graduate degree in another field. This is often an option for those who want to study nursing as a second career. These are people who are clear about their nursing career goals, have investigated their options carefully, and are looking for the most facilitative path to achieve them.

The program composition varies from school to school; some may be completed in four semesters, including one semester that requires a five-day-a-week, three-month-long clinical internship. Like students in accelerated BSN programs, students enrolling in these programs need to be prepared for an intellectually and physically demanding educational challenge. For additional information about these programs, including a comprehensive list of accelerated master's programs, see the AACN *Issue Bulletin* entitled "Accelerated Programs: The Fast-Track to Careers in Nursing" at *www.aacn.nche.edu/publications/issues/Aug02.htm.*

The Clinical Nurse Leader (CNL)

The Clinical Nurse Leader was created by AACN to meet the growing concerns and complexities of healthcare delivery including the nursing shortage, patient safety issues, and other emerging healthcare challenges. Although prepared at the master's level, the CNL is not considered an advanced practice role, although it has been compared to the clinical nurse specialist. To read about the differences and similarities of these roles, log on to *www.aacn.org* and find your way to "Working Statement Comparing the Clinical Nurse Leader and the Clinical Nurse Specialist Roles: Differences Similarities and Complementarities." Many college and university nursing programs are offering master's level degrees as CNLs. Employment opportunities are emerging. Those interested in this degree would be wise to familiarize themselves with information about the role, including the pros, cons, available positions, and controversy raised in dialogues among the faculty and leadership of the professional nursing community.

The Doctoral Degree in Nursing

Doctoral programs prepare nurses to expand and contribute to nursing knowledge through scholarly work, research, advanced practice, nursing/healthcare administration, and/or teaching. A doctorally prepared nurse is an influential leader who can have roles in a variety of healthcare and academic settings (e.g., as a nurse executive leading the nursing division and its related healthcare services in a major medical center or as the dean and/or tenured professor in a university-based college of nursing program).

Educational Preparation

The doctoral degrees that are typically granted include the following:

- **PhD:** Doctor of Philosophy
- **EdD:** Doctor of Education
- **DNSc or DNS:** Doctor of Nursing Science
- **DNP:** Doctor of Nursing Practice. This is a new degree credential based on the work of AACN's Roadmap Task Force, which is recommending that by 2015, this "practice doctorate be the graduate degree for advanced nursing practice preparation, including but

not limited to the four current advanced practice nursing roles: clinical nurse specialist, nurse anesthetist, nurse midwife, and nurse practitioner." You can read more about and track the unfolding events related to this important issue at *www.aacn.nche.edu/dnp/pdf/DNProadmapreport.pdf.*

DISTANCE OR ONLINE LEARNING PROGRAMS

As familiarity with the computer and the Internet increase, and high-speed communication links among people become more commonplace and indispensable, traditional face-to-face education is being supplemented or, in some cases, replaced with online learning in virtual rather than "brick-and-mortar" classrooms. Students, including those in nursing programs, increasingly have the option of online as well as traditional education courses and programs. *Online education, distance learning,* and *distance education* are the terms used to describe the learning that occurs in classrooms that are virtual rather than real.

In its online publication called "Distance Education: A Consumer's Guide," the Western Cooperative for Educational Telecommunications (WCET) defines *distance education* as

> instruction that occurs when the instructor and student are separated by distance or time, or both. A wide array of technologies is currently being used to link the instructor and student. Courses are offered via videotape, broadcast television, ITFS (Instructional Television Fixed Service), microwave, satellite, interactive video, audio tapes, audio-conferencing, CD-ROM, and increasingly, networking—including email, the Internet, and its World Wide Web.

This guide is a very helpful resource for those contemplating online education and can be accessed at *www.wcet.info/resources/publications/conguide/conguida.htm.* In addition, you may find the following websites useful: *www.elearners.com/guide/why-online-education/you-are-ready-to-go-back-to-school-if/* and *www.distance-learning-college-guide.com/.* The exploration of the following topics will allow you to assess thoroughly your readiness for this type of learning, including how to get started:

- Who are distance learners?
- Where do I begin?
- How do I choose a school?
- How do I evaluate quality?
- What is accreditation?

- Even if a school is accredited, how do I make sure it's electronically offered programs are of high quality?
- How do I evaluate a program from a school that is not accredited? (I highly suggest that you do not attend a school that is not accredited, because it may interfere with opportunities for financial aid and/or future educational programs' recognition of your degree.)
- What is the best technology to use?
- Making a decision
- Resources on the Internet

According to WCET's guide, students who enroll in distance-learning courses require the skills and attributes listed below. Place a check mark next to the ones you believe you have:

- ❐ Good time management skills
- ❐ Self-motivation and discipline
- ❐ Comfort with using a computer
- ❐ Flexible learning styles
- ❐ Motivation

Those who participate in online learning programs will need access to and familiarity with the following computer-based tools: email, listservs, discussion groups, chat rooms, streaming video, desktop videoconferencing, and websites. The use of these tools will vary, depending on the type of online program you select. Distance-learning courses are highly interactive experiences with direct access to teachers and classmates through email communication. They contain the same objectives, workload, assignments, and expectations as classroom options, except that the student can choose the time of day and for how long to attend the virtual class to fulfill the requirements. The clinical practice component, if required, is taught close to the student's home by qualified nurse preceptors at local healthcare organizations, which are chosen carefully and evaluated by the degree-granting institution. This kind of choice and control in relation to time management makes distance education an extremely attractive option for busy nurses.

CONTINUING EDUCATION

The educational preparation of degree-granting programs (BSN, master's, etc.) arms the nurse with basic information and provides a foundation upon which to build a nursing practice. Ongoing continuing education (CE) ensures that this information stays current so that nursing skills and competencies are effectively and safely employed.

A lifelong commitment to professional education is not only a hallmark of the professional nurse but extremely important in light of rapidly changing and emerging technologies, as well as the explosion of discoveries in health and science. It also ensures that the mind-set and attitude of the nurse changes and develops over time, an essential characteristic for nurses who seek to influence others and build relationships in their work.

While continuing education is the nurse's professional and ethical responsibility, it is also frequently mandated for license renewal by the boards of nursing of each state. Since CE requirements differ greatly from state to state, nurses must keep track of the current or changing requirements of the state in which they are practicing. Each of the state nurses' associations or the state boards of nursing provide this information at their websites or in writing upon request. An additional way to determine what your requirements might be is through one of the nursing-specific sites that provides career information, such as Nurse.com (*www.nurse.com*).

For nurses who are board certified by the American Nurses Credentialing Center (ANCC) or by nursing specialty associations, continuing education along with a specified number of practice hours is mandatory for recertification. This information can be obtained at ANCC's website (*www.nursecredentialing.org*) and at the websites of the specialty associations through which you are certified.

Some organizations that offer continuing education programs are the following:

- **Nursing Center** (*www.nursingcenter.com*). Select your own CE topic using the site's search engine. Offerings include the following:
    - Outcomes Research: An Interdisciplinary Perspective
    - Right Ventricular Myocardial Infarction: When Power Fails
    - Diversity Issues in the Delivery of Healthcare
- **New York State Nurses Association** (*www.nysna.org*). Offerings include these:
    - Preventing Medication Errors
    - End of Life Care
    - Domestic Violence: The Nurse's Role

- **Stony Brook University School of Nursing** (*www.nursing.stonybrook.edu*). Select your CE topic of interest using the search engine. Offerings include these:
  - Cost Analysis in the Healthcare Arena
  - Infant Security in the Maternal and Pediatric Settings
  - Helping Nurses Publish in Nursing Journals
- **Nurse.com** (*www.nurse.com*). Offerings include the following:
  - Abdominal Aortic Aneurysm
  - Earning Degrees by Distance Education
  - Psychiatric Nursing in Correctional Settings
- **RnCeus.com** (*www.rnceus.com*). Offerings include these:
  - Hormones in Pregnancy
  - Understanding Coagulation Tests
  - Biochemical Terrorism: An Emergency Room Resource

To explore many more of these options, type "online nursing education" into any search engine (refer to chapter 4). Search engines that are nursing-specific will provide you with many lists of CE programs. Nursing-specific search engines can be found at *www.ultimatenurse.com, www.nursing.advanceweb.com, www.nurse.com,* and *www.nursingworld.org.*

CONTINUING THE JOURNEY

Lucille Joel, RN, EdD, FAAN, a renowned nursing leader and educator, believes a long-standing problem in the nursing profession that erodes the professional image of the registered nurse is that "nurses have traditionally derived their identity from their statutory title, RN, rather than from their academic preparation."

Committing yourself to lifelong nursing education in all its variations ensures the strength of your nursing identity and your readiness for the opportunities and challenges of the 21st century.

CHAPTER 4

The Nurse and Information Technology

> The constant dilemma of the information age is that our ability to gather a sea of data greatly exceeds the tools and techniques available to sort, extract and apply the information we've collected.
>
> —*Jeff Davidson, author of* Breathing Space

> Science and technology multiply around us. To an increasing degree, they dictate the languages in which we speak and think. Either we use those languages, or we remain mute.
>
> —*J. G. Ballard, novelist*

Throughout your nursing career, you will be utilizing many methods of information technology. Regardless of the setting, whether an intensive care unit, a medical-surgical unit, the operating room, a home care setting, or an outpatient clinic, information technology offers real improvements for patients, the ability to streamline documentation, and a way to facilitate communication among the interdisciplinary team. The new nursing specialty of nursing informatics provides today's nurse with a resource person and ally as well as a potential career path.

This chapter will assist you in strengthening your relationship with some of the information technology common in nursing practice and provide you with an overview of its ubiquitous presence and influence. It is important to remember that while information technology *assists* nurses in the delivery of patient care, it should never be considered a *replacement* for the nurse's education and experience; critical thinking skills and judgment remain essential components required for excellence in patient care.

Consider how the following features, components, and flow of information technology benefit today's patient care delivery:

- **Data Collection:** Information that was previously collected on paper can now be entered into electronic systems through a variety of input devices, including desktop computers, laptops, handheld devices, or input from other computer systems. The goal is to enter the data once and share as needed with multiple computer applications. Not only does this prevent repeatedly asking the same questions of patients and families, it also works toward getting essential data such as allergies and medication histories to other healthcare providers in a timely and accurate manner.

- **Data Storage:** Collected data can be stored in a variety of applications and transferred to other applications as needed.
- **Data Communication and Sharing Between Systems:** Different computer systems store data and are programmed to send these data to other systems as needed. Only relevant information is shared, and protections are put in place to ensure the safety and confidentiality of the stored data.
- **Patient Care:** Information technology enables the nurse to gather information such as laboratory results, patient histories, and nursing care plans from electronic systems. They can also enter vital information into these systems, making it available to other members of the healthcare team.
- **Data Mining and Research:** Healthcare providers can gather specific data from the wealth of stored information now available to provide safe and effective patient care and to conduct studies to evaluate and improve patient care. In addition, computers generate the reports required by regulatory agencies, insurance companies, and other appropriate entities in a timelier manner than do paper systems.
- **Patient Education and Staff Development:** At their place of employment, nurses can access prepared patient education materials from hospital data systems. At work or at home, they can log on to approved continuing education sites sponsored by nursing organizations or through online journals.
- **Quality Monitoring and Improvement:** Stored data can be available to conduct quality monitoring and improvement projects, allowing changes in patient care to occur more rapidly.

TECHNOLOGY HAS CHANGED HEALTHCARE

Many nurses practicing today were witnesses to the technological explosion in the healthcare workplace that started in small ways, such as the digital thermometers that replaced the glass and mercury versions and intravenous pumps that electronically monitored infusion rates. More and more complicated and sophisticated electronic tools and machinery have embedded themselves into the fabric of healthcare delivery. Specialized care emerged in response to more and more patients being tethered to computerized equipment. Intensive care units challenged nurses to combine familiar high-touch skills with new high-tech ones.

Technology changed procedures like cardiac catheterization and many others. Sonograms allowed a much improved view into interior body spaces. Computed tomography scans, positron emission tomography scans, and magnetic resonance imaging revealed even more information, allowing faster and more precise diagnoses and treatment. Laser and laparoscopic surgery replaced a lot of traditional surgical procedures, allowing patients to go home sooner, less sick, and with faster recovery periods.

This may sound like ancient history to younger generations of nurses, but the 25 years or so that it has taken for technology to transform healthcare is hardly enough to qualify as ancient.

DAILY ENCOUNTERS WITH TECHNOLOGY

Today's nurse is technologically proficient, computer literate, and Internet savvy. She or he is ready and willing to master the technology required, understand the potential obsolescence of it, and adapt to what's new and what's next. To get a glimpse into how technology has infiltrated today's nursing practice, let's follow Ida and Sam, two medical-surgical nurses, for part of their workday. How similar are their activities to yours? Or to how you would like to work?

Technology in Practice by Two Nurses: Ida and Sam

Ida and Sam use the hospital's computer systems to communicate with and send information to the hospital's various departments and to other members of the healthcare team.

Upon entry by a licensed prescriber, an order is immediately printed out as a request in the radiology department, pharmacy, or laboratory, allowing Sam and Ida more time to focus on patient care issues. Bar-coded information is returned with the lab results or medication, reducing the chance of error.

Ida uses the computer at the bedside and/or the nursing station for entering documentation on her patients and to obtain prior medical records. She is pleased with how quickly she can access information that once took so much more time. Gone are the forms to fill out and the calls to request medical records. Her friend Barbara is a psychiatric home care nurse and uses a laptop with dropdown menus to check off appropriate words related to the patient's status rather than writing long paragraphs. Barbara also uses specialized software to schedule patients for office and clinic visits, treatments, and surgery, bragging about how much time she saves by doing it this way.

Sam has been teaching a newly diagnosed diabetic patient how to give himself insulin injections and is pleased to see how much the patient learned from the three online diabetic education sites he encouraged the patient to explore. This patient is an Internet enthusiast and told Sam about many other sites that he found, some of which had different information than Sam had given him. Sam used this opportunity to caution the patient about carefully critiquing the many sites he'll find when surfing the Web, especially if he is reading a research study. He told the patient to use the following questions to determine the accuracy of the data: How current is the information? What are the credentials of the person or organization offering the information? How large was the research study, and were the results duplicated anywhere? He gave the patient the following healthcare websites that could be trusted to provide accurate and up-to-date information:

- Mayo Clinic: *www.mayoclinic.com*
- U.S. Department of Health and Human Services, Office of Disease Prevention and Health Promotion: *www.healthfinder.gov*
- The American Heart Association: *www.americanheart.org*
- The National Institutes of Health: *www.nih.gov*
- The American Diabetic Association: *www.diabetes.org*

Sam also showed this patient how to use email to contact a list of health providers specializing in diabetes that have home pages filled with good information. Sam was pleased to hear that the patient's health insurance company had already registered him for its health-oriented email services.

Sam and Ida both use the hospital's Internet access to use reference tools and research-oriented websites and have come to rely on these to support an evidence-based approach to nursing practice. Neither of them can imagine getting along without the Internet now. Some of Sam and Ida's favorite clinical reference tools appear in the "Clinical Reference Tools" box below.

Sam and Ida's Clinical Reference Tools

- Lippincott's Nursing Center: *www.nursingcenter.com/home/index.asp*
- Online Journal of Issues in Nursing: *www.nursingworld.org/ojin*
- Auscultation Assistant (hear actual heart and breath sounds): *wilkes.med.ucla.edu/intro.html*
- Medlineplus: *medlineplus.gov*
- RxList: *www.rxlist.com*
- The Cochrane Collection: *cochrane.org*

Sam and Ida are each on different committees related to the hospital's information technology (IT) initiatives. Sam is working with the IT department to revise the electronic medical records. Ida is one of the nursing representatives on the privacy and confidentiality program committee, which explores methods to maintain the security of data stored in the patient's hospital record. Ida is enjoying the ability to use her long-standing interest and experience in patient advocacy. She will be participating in the staff education program about issues related to maintaining the confidentiality of patient information, including the federal regulations enacted to protect the patient's privacy. This program will also address the importance of storing codes and passwords used to log on to computer programs in a safe, confidential manner.

Both Sam and Ida are pleased to be able to provide patients with a computer printout of discharge instructions, including medication directions, a duplicate of which remains in the patient's computerized record.

Recently, Sam shared his career goal with Ida. He was investigating graduate nursing programs that prepared informatics nurses. He felt sure that combining his interest in and knack for technology with his growing nursing competence would make for a very satisfying career option.

THE INTERNET: THE OTHER HEALTHCARE REVOLUTION

Accessing and using information, the currency of these times, as well as staying connected to others through high-speed communication devices, have changed the way we live and work. As a user of these devices, you are likely to be familiar with the following commonly used terms.

- **Internet:** A vast array of separate networks that are maintained by individuals or organizations that are linked together, acting as a kind of unified whole for the purpose of sharing, transmitting, and communicating news, information, and services. It is important to remember that what you post on the Internet is potentially available for uninvited others to see. Select a different means of communication if privacy is a primary concern. Be sure to utilize secure sites, especially where identifiable patient information is concerned. Refer to chapter 12 ("The Networking Department of *You, Inc.*") for additional discussion related to ensuring patient privacy and confidentiality. Safeguarding your own identifying information (Social Security and credit card numbers, for example) is also essential.
- **Intranet:** An intranet is an agency- or employer-specific network that is used for employee communication and transmission of documents. Because it is employer owned, anything you post of a personal, confidential nature and all websites you access may be tracked and viewed by the employer. For this reason, be cautious about your use of the Intranet for non-work-related reasons.
- **Search engine:** A program that searches documents for specific keywords and returns a list of these documents to the requester. Google and Yahoo! are examples of search engines.
- **Blog:** A blog is a web-based log that allows you to create a commentary of response to a particular topic; a blog may have a running list of comments from others. Blogs are popular and used extensively in professional, business, and political communities. Refer to chapter 12 ("The Networking Department of *You, Inc.*") for additional discussions about the use of blogs in nursing.
- **Listserv:** An automatic mailing list server. Email is addressed to a Listserv mailing list and then broadcast to everyone who subscribes to the list. This results in a newsgroup or forum, a kind of online community of people with particular an interests.
- **Email:** Short for electronic mail, it is the transmission of messages over the Internet or an intranet.

INTERNET RESOURCES

The Internet has become an important and indispensable tool for your nursing practice and in the management of your career. A sampling of the vast Internet resources that can be accessed appear below, divided into the following categories of interest to nurses: professional practice, nursing research, nursing education, employment/career management, and nursing community. This is not meant to be an all-inclusive list but rather to provide you with examples of what is available. See Resources at the back of the book for additional recommendations.

Professional and Clinical Practice

There is a vast number of national and international nursing organizations, associations, and institutions to which you can connect and with whom you can interact to enhance your professional growth, track important professional practice issues, and access clinical information useful to evidence-based practice.

One of the many ways to find lists of and links to nursing and healthcare sites is to access the website of the American Nurses Association (ANA) at *www.nursingworld.org*. The ANA reports on national nursing issues, provides resources related to clinical nursing practice, discusses actions of government agencies, and more. These reports and articles will include links to additional websites of interest, where you will find even more links moving you onward into cyberspace. ANA sites include the following:

- Academic organizations
- General nursing practice forums and institutes
- International nursing organizations
- Listservs and newsgroups
- Publications and references
- Specialty practice associations
- State boards of nursing index
- Online continuing education

Examples of other sites that will provide you with similar information include these:

- Pennsylvania State Nurses Association *www.panurses.org*
- New York State Nurses Association *nysna.org/links.htm*
- Nursing Spectrum *www.nurse.com*
- Advance for Nurses *nursing.advanceweb.com/main.aspx*

Additional sites of interest to professional and clinical practice include the following:

- **The National Institutes of Health (NIH)** ***www.nih.gov*** Offers information about healthcare, research, grants, diseases, clinical trials, and so on. Examples of what you might find on the NIH homepage include information about the West Nile Virus and hormone replacement therapy.
- **The Centers for Disease Control and Prevention (CDC)** ***www.cdc.gov*** This federal agency protects the health and safety of people in the United States by monitoring health in the nation and in the world. Examples of what you would find at the CDC homepage include the use of the smallpox vaccine and information about anthrax.
- **The Food and Drug Administration (FDA)** ***www.fda.gov*** This federal agency provides health and safety through the regulation of food, cosmetics, medical devices, and so on. An example of what you might find at this site is information about buying medications online.
- **The International Council of Nurses (ICN)** ***www.icn.ch*** Represents nurses from 120 countries. Its mission is to provide quality nursing practice and influence health policy. Issues of interest you will find at this site include AIDS and primary healthcare.
- The mission of the **World Health Organization (WHO),** ***www.who.int/en,*** is to monitor the health needs of people worldwide. Health issues you will find at this site include communicable diseases, traveler health needs, and so on.
- At the site of the **American Medical Association (AMA),** ***ama-assn.org,*** you can track issues related to medical practice as well as it's relationship with other healthcare disciplines and healthcare concerns in general.
- Issues of relevance to nursing practice can often be found in **JAMA, the *Journal of the American Medical Association, jama.ama-assn.org*,** including an important study about the nursing shortage

conducted by Peter Buerhaus, PhD, RN, of Vanderbilt University and his colleagues from Dartmouth that has been available to read online as of June 2002.

- To track licensure issues online, access the website of the **National Council for State Boards of Nursing** at *ncsbn.org*. Because each state has different nurse practice and regulation acts, this site will guide you through the use of its search engine to the state in which you require information.
- **Nursing publications and resources of interest to nurses** can be accessed at *www.nursingnet.org*. Here you will find links to national and international journals, publications, and reference tools, including the National Library of Medicine, *Medscape*, *Medline*, *The Merck Manual*, and many, many more.

NURSING RESEARCH

For news on research, abstracts, poster sessions, and other research-oriented information, access the websites of state nurses associations (for example, the New York State Nurses Association at *www.nysna.org*) and find the link to "nursing research." Other nursing associations, such as the Eastern Nursing Research Society at *www.enrs.org*, will provide similar information. Also access Sigma Theta Tau, International Honor Society of Nursing (*nursingsociety.org*), and find the link to the Florence Henderson International Library. Dissertation abstracts are available online from many schools, including Barry University at *barry.edu/nursing/PHD/disertationAbstracts.htm*. You will find other electronic resources, such as the CDC at *www.cdc.gov* and The Cochrane Collection at *www.cochrane.org*, important sources of information to support your inquiries about clinical questions and evidence-based nursing practice.

ONLINE NURSING EDUCATION

Many colleges, universities, and other approved institutions and organizations offer continuing education, courses required for degree completion, and entire degree programs online as distance-learning options.

Graduate programs in such specialties as nursing informatics are ever increasing. Several test preparation sites, such as *www.kaptest.com*, are useful for nursing students preparing for state board licensing exams. This site will also link you to information about other tests, including the Graduate Record Examination (GRE), which is often required for graduate school entry.

For continuing education, often a requirement for relicensure and professional certification, try the website of your state nurses association. Refer to chapter 3 ("Nursing Education") for additional discussion of online learning options.

EMPLOYMENT AND CAREER MANAGEMENT

Many local and national sites can be accessed to explore employment possibilities. Among them are these:

- Monster.com *www.monster.com*
- Nursing Spectrum *www.nursingspectrum.com*
- American Nurses Association *www.nursingworld.org*
- Career Builder *www.careerbuilder.com*

Also try the website of any healthcare organization in which you are interested in seeking employment. Use search engines to locate the organizations of interest and then find links to their human resources departments.

For assistance writing your resumes and cover letters, try these sites:

- Career Journal *jobstar.org*
- Monster.com *career-advice.monster.com*
- Kaplan Career Center *www.kaptest.com*

For interview practice using virtual interview questions, log on to Monster.com: *career-advice.monster.com*

For tips on how to prepare for job fairs, go to *jobsearch.about.com/library/blfairtip.htm.*

NURSING COMMUNITY

One way in which you can stay connected to colleagues in the local, national, and international nursing community is by utilizing listservs and usenet newsgroups. Explore the ones provided below and find more on your own.

Listservs (Also Called Email Lists)

- *www.nurse.com*
- *www.nursingspectrum.com/nursecommunity/index.htm*
- *nursingworld.org* for lists of listservs maintained by the ANA

Usenet Newsgroups

These are available on Internet service providers such as America Online (AOL) and through any search engine when investigating a particular interest. For example, if you are a nursing student and want information related to the NCLEX-RN® exam, from any search engine, type in "NCLEX test prep" and among the many sites that will appear, you will find the Kaplan Test Prep Center. Following the links, you will eventually be led to a site for *The Nursing Edge*, an email newsletter about the NCLEX RN® exam and other information to plan and advance your nursing career.

THE INFORMATICS NURSE: A SPECIALITY IN GREAT DEMAND

The role of nursing informatics emerged within the last few decades as the use of computer-based data and the Internet became omnipresent in healthcare delivery. This nursing specialty is an essential member of healthcare teams nationwide responding to the push from multiple agencies, including the federal and state governments, to convert patients' medical records to a completely electronic system.

In 2008, the ANA defined the scope of practice for nursing informatics, nursing science, computer science, and information science as being to manage and communicate data, information, knowledge, and wisdom in nursing practice. Nursing informatics supports consumers, patients, nurses, and other providers in their decision making in all roles and settings. This support is accomplished through the use of information structures, information processes, and information technology.

Many nursing and other multiprofessional groups are available for nurses interested in informatics. Listed below are a few of them.

- ANIA-CARING
  www.ania-caring.org

The purpose of ANIA-CARING (formerly the American Nursing Informatics Association and the Capital Area Roundtable on Informatics in Nursing) is to advance the field of nursing informatics through communication, education, research, and professional activities. Its mission is to provide education, networking, and information resources that enrich and strengthen the roles in the field of nursing informatics.

- American Health Information Management Association (AHIMA)
  www.ahima.org

AHIMA is the premier association of health information management professionals. AHIMA's more than 60,000 members are dedicated to the effective management of personal health information required to deliver quality healthcare to the public. Founded in 1928 to improve the quality of medical records, AHIMA is committed to advancing the health information management profession in an increasingly electronic and global environment through leadership in advocacy, education, certification, and lifelong learning.

- Health Information and Management Systems Society (HIMSS)
  www.himss.org/ASP/index.asp

HIMSS is a cause-based, not-for-profit organization exclusively focused on providing global leadership for the optimal use of information technology and management systems for the betterment of healthcare.

- American Medical Informatics Association (AMIA)
  www.amia.org

AMIA is dedicated to promoting the effective organization, analysis, management, and use of information in healthcare in support of patient care, public health, teaching, research, administration, and related policy. AMIA's 4,000 members advance the use of health information and communications technology in clinical care and clinical research, personal health management, public health/population, and translational science with the ultimate objective of improving health.

AMIA is an interdisciplinary and diverse group of individuals and organizations that come from over 65 countries. Individual members include the following:

- Physicians, nurses, dentists, pharmacists, and other clinicians
- Researchers and educators
- Advanced students pursuing a career in informatics

- Scientists and developers
- Government officials and policy makers
- Consultants and industry representatives
- Standards developers

There is also a very informative journal: *CIN: Computers Informatics Nursing.*

It could be said that the first informatics nurse was Florence Nightingale according to Linda Thede in her book, *Informatics and Nursing* (2003). She draws the following lineage from the 19th century to the 21st century:

> Recognizing the value of data in affecting healthcare, during her service in the nineteenth century war in the area of Russia called the Crimea, she collected data and systematized record-keeping practices. Using these data, she developed the pie graph to dramatize the need for reform to stop the needless deaths caused by unsanitary conditions in military hospitals.
>
> With the advent of the computer, the use of data is far more widespread than it was in Nightingale's time. When decisions are based on the data available, the need for the collection and analysis of nursing data become very important. Without nursing data, the value of nursing will continue to be hidden to many people in policy-making positions. Through nursing informatics, the healthcare information systems that are being developed will include the nursing data needed to show the value that nurses add to healthcare.

These nursing data which include information about the patient, institutional information, domain knowledge (knowledge of nursing and other disciplines), and procedural knowledge provide the basis for evidence based practice. Informatics is the specialty responsible for synthesizing these data sources into a workable whole for the use by healthcare practitioners (Thede, 2003).

Educational preparation for the informatics nurse is achieved by obtaining a master's level degree specializing in nursing informatics, completing certificate programs, or engaging in on-the-job training. The number of programs is ever increasing. The best programs are the ones that require students to have clinical experiences working alongside a nurse informatics specialist. Look for programs that emphasize a philosophy in which students are reminded that they are always nurses first and informatics specialists next.

The American Nurses Credentialing Center, the arm of the ANA that provides certification in many nursing specialties, offers certification for the informatics nurse who meets the following qualifications:

- Holds a current, active RN license in a state or territory of the United States or the professional, legally recognized equivalent in another country.
- Has practiced the equivalent of two years full-time as an RN.
- Holds a baccalaureate or higher degree in nursing or a baccalaureate degree in a relevant field.
- Has completed 30 hours of continuing education in informatics within the last three years.
- Meets one of the following practice hour requirements:
  - Has a practiced minimum of 2,000 hours in informatics nursing within the last three years.
  - Has practiced a minimum of 1,000 hours in informatics nursing in the last three years and has completed a minimum of 12 semester hours of academic credit in informatics courses that are a part of a graduate-level informatics nursing program.
  - Has completed a graduate program in nursing informatics containing a minimum of 200 hours of faculty-supervised practicum in informatics.

The multiple roles in which the informatics nurse might be practicing are included in the following list.

POSSIBLE ROLE	RESPONSIBILITES
Project manager	Plans and implements an informatics project; communicates effectively with all levels of management, users, and systems developers; is familiar with managing change, assessing need for new projects, planning and implementation.
Systems specialist	Acts as link between nursing and information services as a nursing resource and representative.
Consultant	Provides expert advice, opinions, and recommendations utilizing nursing expertise; analyzes client needs, technologically and organizationally; may be employed by organization vendor or be self-employed.

Systems educator	Provides training in information systems, including new systems; orientation of new employees; and train-the-trainer programs.
Systems analyst/ developer	Participates in the development of new information systems, including designing informatics solutions to nursing problems; understands the needs of nursing.
Policy developer	Contributes to healthcare policy development by identifying nursing data related to information management, healthcare, and economics.
Entrepreneur	Analyzes nursing information needs in clinical areas, education, administration, and research; develops and markets solutions.

SUMMARY

The opportunities afforded by informatics in nursing and healthcare range from improving patient care through making our professional lives easier, to recognition of the value that nursing adds to healthcare. Like all opportunities, these will not be reached without meeting the challenges of working with information and adopting it to nursing, rather adapting nursing to the needs for information.

Nursing information is not solely the province of nursing informatics specialists, all nurses must be involved if successful information systems are to be developed and implemented.

—Linda Q. Thede[1]

CHAPTER 5

The Newly Graduated Nurse

WELCOME TO NURSING!

> The future belongs to those who believe in the beauty of their dreams.
>
> —*Eleanor Roosevelt*

Now that you've graduated, it's time to start on the next phase of your journey in becoming a nurse. You are embarking on a career in which you will be able to take advantage of experiences that are among the finest opportunities for professional and personal growth to be found anywhere. You've made a great choice!

You are entering the profession at an important time: exciting new roles are emerging, and potentially transformative changes are occurring in workplace policies and programs aimed at increasing nurse satisfaction. These changes are driven by many factors, including attempts to mitigate the nursing shortage through the redesign of the workplace to make it more possible for mature nurses to continue working rather than retire. Employer practices under scrutiny and targeted for revision include nurse-to-patient staffing ratios and mandatory overtime policies, both sources of long-standing discord and stress for all nurses.

This is a time of turning points and crossroads, a time when some of the old ways that have limited and distorted the image and value of nursing are beginning to fade. Having a positive perception of these changes can shape your purpose, clarify your mission, and enhance the vision of yourself as a nurse, ultimately providing you with the professional satisfaction you are seeking.

Think back to the image you had of yourself as a nurse before entering nursing school—what you imagined you would be doing, how, where, and with whom. Now, fast-forward to the image you currently have of yourself. Is it the same? Is it different?

Most likely, the experiences you had and the people you met as you moved through your years of school have modified but not entirely changed the ideal image you might have had, replacing it with an image far closer to reality. This same process of moving from the ideal to the real is about to happen all over again as you leave the familiar nursing school community and enter the nursing practice workplace. Your challenge will be to adapt to the reality of the work world without leaving all of your ideals and values behind.

You've most likely left nursing school with a certain sense of mastery and proficiency about how to be a nursing student, along with an accumulation of knowledge that now needs to be applied so that you can develop the skills and competencies that will eventually define you as a nurse. In your first job, your nursing identity will start to emerge, fragile at first but hopefully protected and nurtured by the guidance and mentoring of those who came before you, while they also permit enough space for your unique nursing personality to bloom.

THE JOURNEY FROM NOVICE TO EXPERT

To be a new graduate is to straddle two worlds, the recent past and the hopeful future, while maneuvering through what might feel like an obstacle course of learning challenges. Upon beginning work, you will be considered a novice or an advanced beginner (see figure 5.1) and move through five progressive stages that, over the years and after accumulated experience, will qualify you as an expert nurse. You might already be familiar with this learning model, developed by Patricia Benner, RN, PhD, FAAN, and described in her book *From Novice to Expert*.[1] Refreshing your memory about these stages can reassure you about what to expect and provide you with guideposts that will help you chart your course and measure your progress.

J. Mae Pepper, PhD, RN, in her book *Conceptual Bases of Professional Nursing*,[2] adapted Benner's five stages, as described on page 72.

Keep in mind that these stages are fluid; a change in specialties or roles may require deskilling and reskilling and a transit through these stages once more. So having patience with yourself is essential. Crucial to your ability to cope with the transition from student to nurse is a realistic understanding of the time lines of these stages. While there are exceptions, the average time spent in these stages is as follows:

- Two to three years in the same setting to achieve the competence of Stage III
- An additional year or so to achieve the proficiency of Stage IV
- An extensive and undetermined number of years to achieve the expert status of Stage V

	Stage I	Stage II	Stage III	Stage IV	Stage V
Title	Novice*	Advanced Beginner	Competent	Proficient	Expert
Experience Level	Pre-graduate*	New Graduate	2–3 years in the same setting	3–5 years	Extensive
Character-istics of Performance	—Is flexible	—Formulates principles	—Plans	—Perceives "wholes"	—Has an intuitive grasp
	—Exhibits rule-governed behaviors	—Needs help with priority setting	—Feelings of mastery	—Interprets nuances	

* Stage I (the novice stage) occurs in nursing school. The newly graduated nurse begins nursing practice at Stage II, the advanced beginner.

Figure 5.1 Benner's Stages from Novice to Expert Nurse

TRANSITIONING INTO A NEW REALITY

New graduates straddle two worlds: the familiar world of nursing school and the not so familiar world of nursing practice. It can feel very disquieting to think you have to abandon school values and adopt work values with which you may not fully agree. Marlene Kramer coined a term for this and titled her book with it: *Reality Shock* (1977). In this seminal work, she explores the role of conflict in this critical transitional experience and says reality shock happens when

> newcomers in an occupational field find themselves in a work situation for which they have spent several years preparing and for which they thought they were going to be prepared, and then suddenly find that they are not.

It soon becomes evident to the newcomer that the professional ideals and values learned in school are not fully operational nor are they totally embraced or accepted by those in the workplace. This conflict in values is necessary to resolve if the newcomer is to make a successful transition. Kramer's four stages through which new graduates typically move lead to three possible outcomes, as shown on the following page.

Resolution of Reality Shock

Stage I: The Mastery of Skills and Routines

Characteristics:	There is a preoccupation with the development of technical expertise.
Potential conflict:	Fixating on technical skills prevents sufficient focus on learning other aspects of nursing care, such as teaching, emotional support, etc.

Stage II: Social Integration

Characteristics:	Getting along with coworkers and being accepted by them is a major concern.
Potential conflict:	Fear of retaliation and alienation may prevent the new graduate from applying knowledge learned in school.

Stage III: Moral Outrage

Characteristics:	The new graduate feels frustrated and inadequately prepared.
Potential conflict:	New graduates are confused about their role and to what group or individual their loyalty belongs: the healthcare organization, the profession of nursing, or the patient.

Stage IV: Conflict Resolution with Three Possible Outcomes

Outcome #1:	Wholesale rejection of school culture and values leads to a kind of robotic adaptation to work values and behaviors, accompanied by helpless resignation and the potential for burnout.
Outcome #2:	Wholesale rejection of work culture and values leads to job-hopping in the hopes of finding a better match for the school values the new graduate is unwilling to give up; when job-hopping fails, these nurses typically leave the profession altogether or, alternatively, experience hopeless resignation.
Outcome #3:	A joining of school and work cultures; a bicultural compromise solution allows new graduates to use the "best of both worlds" on behalf of the healthcare organization, the patient, and themselves.

It is evident that Outcome #3, a bicultural compromise solution between school and work values, is optimal. Keeping both sets of values in mind as nursing competence and confidence grows over time allows them to be merged in productive and meaningful ways. Nurses who resolve reality shock by opting for either school ideals or workplace practicalities (Outcomes # 1 and 2) will have difficulty finding professional satisfaction. Like the Benner model, this model can provide you with a way to know what to expect so that you can chart your course and measure your progress.

Not only are conflict management skills essential to success in the transition from graduate to nurse, they are also crucial for effective communication and productive team relationships in today's multicultural and intergenerational workplace. Conflict can actually strengthen relationships when disagreements are voiced in nonaggressive ways. Conflict often raises issues that generate creative thought and solutions to problems. Learning to communicate while managing the strong feelings that accompany conflicts will benefit you enormously and allow you to learn and grow—to be changed by the views of others. In the Resources section at the back of this book, you will find suggestions for deepening your understanding and expanding your skills in this crucial area.

THE SECOND-CAREER NURSE

Focused, mature, motivated and committed, eager, possessing a wealth of life experience, fulfilling a childhood dream, wanting to make a difference... These characteristics frequently describe people who choose to make nursing a second career. Many of them are taking a look at nursing for the first time, while others might have needed to delay their nursing career goals earlier in their lives. The selection of nursing as a second career is an increasingly attractive trend for people in their 20s and 30s as compared to earlier times, when most people embarked on nursing education directly from high school. Such factors as the desire to be engaged in meaningful work, unstable economic conditions, and the desire for career security and employability are influencing this decision in the first decade of the 21st century.

According to David Auerbach, principle analyst in the Health and Human Resources Division at the Congressional Budget Office,[4] this surge in older, second-career nurses could potentially offset the projected nursing shortage by reducing the shortfall of new nurses to 340,000 by 2020, far lower than the previously projected shortfall of 760,000 (*www.sciencewatch.com*).

The entry into nursing of this older, second-career nurse has contributed to the increase of the average age of the employed nurse to 46.8 years in 2006, with only 8 percent of RNs under the age of 30, as compared to 26 percent in 1980 (*Americans for Nursing Shortage Relief 2006*).[5] Retention of more mature workers, essential to mitigating the nursing shortage, requires changes in workplace policy and design to accommodate them. You will find a discussion of this issue in chapter 6.

Whatever the reason for their delayed entry into nursing, second-career nurses contribute valuable life and work experience to the nursing workforce, including maturity and transferable skills, such as organization, communication, team collaboration, professionalism, and advanced decision making, They are also experienced in juggling the competing responsibilities of work, family, and personal life.

Profiles of Second-Career Nurses

Tim Hein, Nursing Student

In a 2001 article in the *Business Journal of Milwaukee,*[6] Tim Hein, who was then a 45-year-old RN student, spoke of how he wanted to enter an industry that gave him an opportunity to pursue a hands-on leadership role. He wanted a more versatile degree than the first one he had earned in healthcare management and so chose nursing. The influence of his girlfriend, a nurse, also convinced him it was a good avenue to pursue, even though he wouldn't have considered it 20 years earlier.

Tim believes that the merits of nursing as a second career far outweigh whatever adversities he finds. He says:

> Like anything, nursing takes time. Going back to school is tough, but as a rule, both teachers and students are a helpful group of people. That makes the transition a lot smoother.

Dwight Simmons, Medical-Surgical Nurse

Dwight, age 50, has worked as a nurse for three years and embodies many of the characteristics of second-career nurses. Dwight was an optician for 22 years before he made the transition to nursing, which began 7 years ago after he administered vocational tests to himself and discovered that nursing was one of four careers for which he was best suited. Becoming a nurse, he says, was not a matter of settling. His wife supported the decision and thought he would be great at it.

Dwight correctly assessed the field to be wide open, even though he began nursing school in 1995 at the height of the downsizing and restructuring era in healthcare. Since he already had a degree in biology, he needed only to take the nursing courses, receiving credit for about half of the requirements needed to complete his BSN. He also has an MBA in marketing and one day hopes to follow his nurse manager's (and mentor's) footsteps into management. He envisions himself as a nursing administrator and plans to return to school for a second master's degree, this time in nursing.

In 2004, Dwight was quite content with his experience as a medical-surgical nurse on a liver transplant unit. While a few patients have expressed some surprise and concern about his gender, it is clear that Dwight's comfort with his identity as a nurse eventually puts the patients at ease, while he also models the kind of gender-neutral attitude that nursing needs to embrace. For a discussion about the role of men in nursing, refer to chapter 7. Dwight has the following to say about his nursing experience:

> One of the greatest thrills is when someone comes back to the hospital months later. Sometimes you don't recognize them. You start to cry because they look so wonderful. It makes it all worthwhile.... Being a nurse has given me a better appreciation of life.[7]

Dwight Simmons is certainly on his way to making important contributions to nursing and healthcare. It is clear that he is happy with the decision he made and is a role model for those seeking a second career in nursing.

STRATEGIES FOR SUCCESS

Aim High but Keep Your Expectations Realistic

Every time you become impatient with yourself for not getting something right, every time you think you are taking too long to learn a complex skill or procedure, or whenever you're convinced that you'll never be able to interpret cardiac arrhythmias fast enough, think back to the time line in Benner's stages of proficiencies on page 71, place yourself in it according to the years (not months!) you've been a nurse, and assess yourself accordingly.

Unrealistic expectations of yourself, especially when accompanied by critical or judgmental self-talk, will serve to increase your anxiety, cloud your capacity for critical thinking, influence how you feel about yourself, and eventually affect your ability to master nursing skills and competencies. Consistently holding yourself to a level of proficiency not yet possible creates an obstacle of your own making. Since plenty of obstacles already exist, try not to create more of them. Your emerging nursing identity is vulnerable, and you need to protect it. Allowing yourself to be where you are, not where you wish you could be, combines self-care practice with professional nursing practice. Read more about how self-care is an essential twin partner of your professional development in chapter 15.

Make Use of Mentors and Preceptors

The word *mentor* comes from the Greek legend of Odysseus, who had a loyal friend and wise advisor whose name was Mentor. Establishing a relationship with a mentor is one of the best ways to ensure that your transition from graduate to nurse has the support and nurturing it requires. A mentor is a guide, coach, advocate, role model, and nurturer; a trusted counselor or teacher; a person with whom you establish a relationship for the purpose of helping you to grow professionally and work toward your potential. A mentor might do the following:

- Provide feedback about your performance.
- Assist you in setting and attaining goals, including career planning.
- Identify obstacles to success.
- Empower you to act on your own behalf.

Connie Vance, RN, EdD, FAAN, a professor of nursing at The College of New Rochelle, School of Nursing in New York is author of *The Mentor Connection in Nursing*. She says:

> We all need mentoring—to receive it and to give it—but at particular stages in one's career, it becomes critical. (*www.nurse.com*)[8]

Finding a mentor at this critical time in your career may take some proactive self-direction, but it is worth your time and energy. Perhaps a faculty person would be willing to mentor you, or maybe you'll meet someone suitable at a conference. Or your mentor might be someone who taught in your orientation program. Consider selecting someone who does not work in your unit to ensure objectivity and the ability to speak freely. The Academy of Medical Surgical Nurses has a mentoring program called "Nurses Nurturing Nurses" (N3 for short). It offers two mentoring formats, one hospital based and the other online. Find out more at the website of the Academy of Medical-Surgical Nurses: *www.medsurgnurse.org*.

A mentor can provide an essential reality check and help ensure that potentially inaccurate beliefs do not erode your confidence or negatively influence your nascent nursing identity. At the very minimum, as a new nurse you need a preceptor, someone who acts as a clinical resource while you learn and practice basic nursing skills. Optimally, look for both a mentor and a preceptor. The preceptor will often be assigned to you as part of your orientation program. You may need to find the mentor on your own.

This is a time in nursing that the nurturing inherent in mentoring is needed by everyone. Keep in mind that you don't have to wait until you are at the expert level of nursing proficiency to mentor others in something you are great at and they are not. Read the story of Ida and Sam in chapter 4 to see how they were mentors for one another. You might also want to mentor someone from high school who wants to be a nurse. What an important contribution to the nursing shortage you can make by doing this!

Celebrate Your Achievement

Begin this next phase of your journey on a celebratory note. Just as you met the challenge of nursing school successfully, you can meet these new challenges as well. Remembering this will sustain and encourage you. It is an important foundation of your confidence and self-esteem. Guard it well.

Select Your First Job Carefully

Choices abound. Determine what the expectations will be of you, especially if, because of the nursing shortage, an employer will expect you to function at a level of nursing proficiency sooner than is possible. Get the longest and best orientation possible. Be sure you will have a preceptor; look for a mentor. Ask about the nurse-patient ratio and about staffing and overtime policies. Seek out healthcare employers that have Magnet Status certification for the best nursing practice environments (refer to chapters 1 and 2 for more information about this).

Extend Your Orientation

On your own—that is, after your formal orientation is over—keep it going in any proactive way you can. Explore the continuing education programs in your organization, register for online seminars, and so on. Your graduation from nursing school signaled the continuation of your education, not the end of it.

Be the Best You Can Be

Be kind to yourself as a learner, allowing the time it takes to gain proficiency. Recognize that learning occurs in a process that requires repetition. Forget perfect performance: it doesn't exist anywhere in the universe or within you. As you learn, aim for safety and quality rather than speed, trying not to respond to inner or outer pressures to work faster and do more with less. Much of what you are learning requires practice, practice, practice with a measured dose of patience, patience, patience.

Join a Support Group

Look for a new graduate support group in your organization and join it. Or form one yourself! Seek out mature nurses who are interested in providing their experience and ask them to lead it. Or go online to talk up a storm about what you are experiencing; hear what other nurses think about it and what they are doing. Remember that the stress of many experiences is relieved by the support of others with whom you can talk about common difficulties. You teach this to your patients—now use it for yourself. One online site to explore is *nursezone.com,* where a new-graduate newsletter includes articles, message boards, and blogs. Also check out *www.realityrn.com* for dialogues among new graduates seeking support and advice on such topics as how to present problems to supervisors, how to enlist the help of a seasoned nurse, and the difficulty of delegation.

Seek Out Mature Nurses

An experienced nurse can have a tremendous and lasting impact on your professional life. Mature nurses are typically practicing at the expert level of proficiency and have valuable wisdom and insight to share. They are important clinical and professional resources. This person can often provide you with many decades of nursing history, the spoken, interactive kind you won't find in textbooks or in any other way. The mature nurse represents the brain trust of the nursing profession. You would be wise to tap into this. Recognize that a great strength of the nursing profession is in its cultural and intergenerational diversity, See chapter 6 for an expanded discussion of this topic.

ADVICE FOR SECOND-CAREER NURSES

Getting Started

Keep in mind that to ease the nursing shortage, schools and colleges of nursing are actively recruiting many underrepresented segments of the nursing profession, including men, minorities, and those seeking a second career as a nurse. Look for programs with flexible academic and clinical schedules so that you will be able to accommodate your current needs and responsibilities. Many schools and colleges of nursing have programs specifically designed for second-career nurses. See chapter 3 for additional information on how to select the program that is right for you.

In Nursing School

Give yourself time to adapt to the rigorous academic and clinical learning environment of nursing education. Second-career students may not be prepared for the challenging intensity of nursing education. Nursing school is difficult, and it should be. While communication skills and empathy are a foundation of nursing practice, there is more to being a nurse, including the science of nursing, the mastery of such courses as pathophysiology and pharmacology, and then the application of what you are learning in clinical settings.

Handle the age gap that will most likely exist between you and other students, who could be 10 to 20 or more years younger than you, depending on your own age. Use this as an opportunity to prepare for the intergenerational relationships you will find in nursing practice settings.

To access support and information while in nursing school, use the many wonderful student nurse communities you can find online. One of these is the National Student Nurses' Association (*www.nsna.org*).

In Nursing Practice

Practice balancing the priorities of your work life and your personal life. Refer to chapter 15 for information about why this kind of self-care is essential rather than incidental to your nursing practice.

Temper your enthusiasm with respect and understanding for the first-career nurses with whom you will be working side by side, since this is how you want to be treated as well. Before judging what you may not understand, familiarize yourself with the historic and contemporary influences that impact and shape the variety of responses and behaviors of the profession as well as its individual members. This understanding will pave the way to allowing the contributions you are eager to make be well received.

Just because you're a new graduate doesn't mean you can't make some amazing things happen. One way to do this is to become politically astute and develop relationships in which there can be mutual sharing of ideas, resulting in greater influence and impact. Whether nursing is your first career or your second, whether you are a young nurse or a mature nurse, a woman or a man, you will go far if you are guided by the words of Ralph Waldo Emerson: "*Don't go where the path may lead; go instead where there is no path and leave a trail.*"

CHAPTER 6

The Mature Nurse: Options and Opportunities

> Youth is a gift of nature,
> Age is a work of art.
>
> —*Unknown*
>
> I could not at any age be content to take my place in a corner by the fireside and simply look on.
>
> —*Eleanor Roosevelt*

Across America, the nation's workforce is graying as baby boomers, that large swath of people born between 1946 and 1964, begin to make their exit from the world of work. Compared to earlier generations, this departure, which is taking an atypical path, is not only about to transform the experience of retirement as we know it but stands to make significant changes in the workplace as well. All industries, including healthcare, are gearing up to meet the challenges of this aging workforce.

If healthcare meets these challenges effectively, we can potentially mitigate the nursing shortage as well as improve the working conditions for all nurses that have long contributed to stress and burnout. These conditions include policies associated with unsafe staffing ratios and mandatory overtime, among others.

A longer life span, financial readiness, and labor market influences are among the factors combining at this moment to lead baby boomers (the generation to which most mature nurses belong) to want to work longer or realize they need to. This "longer good-bye," as it was called in a *New York Times* article on retirement, is creating a more gradual winding down, allowing the accumulated knowledge and wisdom of this group to be transferred without leaving as huge and potentially unmanageable a talent void as was expected (*New York Times* 2008).[1]

Concerned with the effects of the loss of this talent and experience, many healthcare organizations and nursing associations are convening conferences, forming think tanks, and conducting surveys in an effort to define the problems associated with the departure of mature nurses, as well as describe the implications and recommend strategies.

In 2005, the Center for American Nurses (CAN) joined the American Association of Retired Persons (AARP) in hosting a roundtable event titled "Workplace of the Future: Spotlight on the Mature Nursing Workforce."[2] This conference addressed "the pressing issues the mature nurses face in the workplace and the challenge of nurse retention as baby boomers retire in growing numbers" (*www.centerforamericannurses.org*). On its website, CAN expresses concern about the necessity to retain mature nurses in the workforce as follows:

> As the Brain Trust of the nursing community, mature nurses are a precious commodity as mentors for younger nurses and are an essential resource of knowledge and experience. Mature nurses present opportunities for informed decision making in creating healthy work environments. (*www.centerforamericannurses.com;* Mature Nurse & Nurse Retention Resources pdf, 2008, page 2.)[3]

A summary of issues and statistics relevant to the mature nursing workforce and to aging workers in general was presented at this conference. These data (tracked by many surveys over the past decade) form the rationale and thrust for the transformative shifts now occurring in the healthcare workplace (2005).

Retention has become the new priority; recruitment has not worked to solve the crisis of the nursing shortage. The revolving-door syndrome is costly to hospitals, with the cost of nurse turnover being approximately $10,000 to $64,000 per nurse (Jones 2004). More than 1 million new and replacement nurses will be needed by 2012 (U.S. Bureau of Labor Statistics 2008–09).[4]

As the nursing workforce ages, the average age for RNs is increasing as follows (Buerhaus, Steiger, & Auerback 2000):

1980	37.9 years
1990	39.5 years
2000	42.1 years
2010	45.4 years (projected)
2020	45.4 years (projected)

Nurses in the under-30 age group predominately work in ICUs, step-down units, labor and delivery units, and emergency departments. The over-50 age group works in operating rooms, postanesthesia care units, general medical-surgical units, outpatient departments, home health agencies, and other nonhospital areas (Buerhaus, Steiger, & Auerback 2000).[5]

The average age of nursing faculty with doctorates in 2001 was 53.2 years with the following age distribution:

Professors	56.2 years
Associate professors	53.8 years
Assistant professors	50.4 years
Master's prepared	49.0 years

The average retirement age in 2001 was 62.5 years. From 2003 to 2012, between 200 and 300 faculty per year will be eligible for retirement (Berlin & Sechrist 2002).[6]

Additional relevant CAN statistics affecting all older workers, including the mature nurse, are as follows:

- One in five Americans ages 55–64 report their health to be only fair or poor. Thirty percent of the 55- to 64-year-old population report having arthritis. One in four men are obese; one in three women are obese.

Older Americans have decreased strength and endurance, manifesting in a degree of difficulty stooping, carrying 25 pounds or more, standing longer than 2 hours, and walking up 10 or more stairs. The older American worker has some cognitive decline, but highly practiced behaviors may be resistant to normal age-related decline. The knowledge base remains intact into advanced age. This group has lower accident rates but stays off work longer if injured; the overall time taken off work is the same as that of younger workers.

WHO IS THE MATURE NURSE?

Considering that nursing workforce is approximately 94 percent female, the mature nurse is likely to be a woman who is a member of the baby boom generation born between 1946 and 1964 or the veteran generation born between 1925 and 1945. A smaller group of nurses were born following World War I and are sometimes referred to as the "lost generation." The actual age of the mature nurse could be as young as 44 or as old as Ardis Martin, who is 96 and still working in 2008! (See her inspiring profile in the following pages.)

A survey of 3,352 mature nurses (all over 40) conducted by the American Nurses Association on its website (Center for American Nurses 2005) revealed additional characteristics of the mature nurse:

- **Number of years in practice:** Years in practice range from 1 to 40 with an average of 23.7 years.

- **Employed in the following settings:**

45.0%	Acute care settings
17.5%	Outpatient settings
15.0%	Educational settings
3.9%	Long-term care
2.9%	Private practice settings, including self-employment

- **Nursing roles:**

40%	Direct care nurses
20%	Nurse managers

- **Educational level:**

35%	Bachelor's-level degree
33%	Master's-level degree
15%	ADN-level degree

- **Degree of work satisfaction:** Of all nurses, 56 percent reported satisfaction. The highest satisfaction was reported by nurses in educational settings or who were self-employed. The lowest level of satisfaction was in acute care or long-term care settings.
- **Reasons nurses think about leaving nursing:**

53%	Mental and emotional stress
44%	Internal/external policies or procedures
47%	Relationships with administration or management
50%	Shift in focus from patient care to finances

It is interesting to note that dissatisfaction with the actual care of patients was not a factor in the decision to retire; rather the dissatisfaction is primarily with management relationships and organizational policies. These data inform the thrust of retention efforts by healthcare organizations. You can read the entire survey by logging on to the publications section of the Center for American Nurses at *www.centerforamericannurses.org*. There you can either purchase the Proceedings Report or download it if you are a member.

PROFILES OF MATURE NURSES

The mature nurse may be on the verge of retiring or is already retired. Those who are retired may be considering a return to work, or they may be very satisfied with a life that no longer has a formal work structure. Alternatively, the mature nurse could be someone who does not plan to retire at all, wanting or needing to continue working on a full-time or part-time basis. It is these nurses (and people like them in other industries) who are part of the cultural redefinition of retirement and who are creating the concept of a "working retirement."

While the focus of this chapter is on issues related to the retention of the mature nurse in the workforce, it seems important to advocate for choice regarding the decision to retire. It is just as appropriate for nurses to decide to retire fully as it is to continue working. That the potential exists for such a choice to be made is a breakthrough shift in American culture, which includes the healthcare industry as well.

In 2001, two nurses who fit the description of the working mature nurse were 61-year-old Marie Cronk and 71-year-old Rosalee Yeaworth (*www.nurseweek.com/news/features/01-01/mature.asp*).[8] At that time Marie, a charge nurse and certified operating room nurse at Good Samaritan Hospital in Puyallup, Washington, was aware of the decline in her physical stamina but said she maintained it effectively through diet and exercise. She also spoke of the value of her experience:

> I feel I have a lot of knowledge and I'm able to use it. And I try to pass it on to the younger people.

Marie's experience encapsulates two important characteristics of the mature nurse. One is to have the option and opportunity to continue contributing and making use of her expertise as a nurse. Mentoring not only meets Marie's needs but those of novice nurses and of the organization. Changes in mental and physical stamina that accompany aging can be managed in part through diet and exercise, as Marie demonstrates. Employers seeking to retain mature nurses are beginning to respond to these physical needs by offering such benefits as gym memberships. This kind of workplace accommodation will be discussed more fully later in this chapter.

Rosalee Yeaworth was a retired dean of the University of Nebraska Medical Center, College of Nursing, and found herself agreeing to teach an Internet course in nursing theory when a faculty member at the college was unable to. She said:

> I went back into teaching last fall not because I needed the money, but because the college needed help. It was stimulating to go back.

Rosalee's desire to return to work as a choice had less to do with a paycheck and more to do with what seemed to be missing in her life without work. She called this missing experience "the need for stimulation." This intangible reward of work could also be called a "sense of purpose" and is often related to the need for community. These important human experiences are what bring people into the nursing profession to begin with. These needs are active over our lifetime, and fulfilling them is just as important in retirement as in a structured work experience.

Marilyn McMahon is another mature nurse. In 2001, at 55, she worked in an emergency room at Forest General Hospital in Hattiesburg, Mississippi. What makes her profile especially interesting is that she worked at the same hospital as her three daughters, also nurses. Their profiles, which appeared in "Bridges Across Time" by Cathryn Domrose in the May 14, 2002,[9] issue of *NurseWeek*, allow a peek into what nurses of different generations can offer one another, as well as what an older nurse still at work might be doing. Mature nurses who have children and grandchildren often want to spend more time with them and state this as a reason to retire. Marilyn has found her own way of spending time with her daughters, as they all work actively as nurses.

Sixty-four-year-old Jacqueline Khan provides us with yet another variation on how mature nurses are working. She entered nursing when she was in her early 50s after a first career as a truant officer with the Detroit Board of Education. She ensured her financial security by staying in that job long enough to qualify for a pension and, while still working, earned her associate's degree in nursing. She "retired" from the Board of Education in 1999 and went back to school for her bachelor's degree in nursing. She is now working 12-hour shifts as a critical care nurse in a level-one trauma hospital in Detroit. Here are a few ways in which Jacqueline describes her experience:

> I want my work to be difficult so I can keep my mind sharp and stay physically fit and all of that .... Inside me is a person who wants to sit down and eat potato chips so I couldn't be in a situation in which that person emerged. I'm going to live my life until it's over. I'm not going to just sit around. I do this for the excitement. I like drama. I like health. I want to be healthy. I don't want to spend my remaining years on this planet not well .... At 64, I really do not think that my life is over; it's still evolving and beginning .... I think I make a direct impact. (Freedman 2007, p.91)[10]

Jacqueline's entry into nursing as a second career provides us with an example of what is contributing to the graying of the nursing workforce, namely that the new graduate is older to begin with. Because she wishes to engage in "difficult work" as a way to keep her mind sharp and keep her body fit (and away from those potato chips!), she is not asking her employer to accommodate her age in ways other mature nurses might want to or need to. Her profile demonstrates the vast diversity and productivity of this group and how valuable a human resource they offer us. More of Jacqueline's story and how she describes the impact she makes as a mature nurse can be found starting on page 90 of Freedman's book, *Encore: Finding Work That Matters in the Second Half of Life* (Freedman, 2007).

And then there is Ardis Martin, who was interviewed by Wendy Bonifazi for the December 2007 issue of *Nursing Spectrum,*[11] in which she was described as "the epitome of a modern nurse." Ardis is 96 years old and still working as the facilitator for the Amarillo Depression and Bipolar Alliance Group in Texas, which she herself started decades ago. While that alone is incredible, so are Ardis's additional achievements. She says about herself as a nurse:

> I became a nurse at age 60, so I've been in nursing only 37 years. I wanted to prove age is not a deterrent to anything you want, and I did it for myself. I was much, much older than most people pursuing a new career, but we've been sold a bill of goods about retiring and loss of competence.

Ardis earned her bachelor's degree in nursing and psychology at age 76 and then her master's in family nursing at age 79. Of this experience she says:

> I retired—or rather resigned—at age 75 so I could go back to school.

It is interesting to note her correction of herself in the use of the words *retired* and *resigned.* More about our current use of the word *retirement* and how it is changing shortly.

Ardis started working in 1930 in a Texas health department lab, but her interest in behavior and why people do what they do led her to become one of the first four people in Texas to earn a mental health degree. Her interest in gerontology and mental health led her to do community outreach in nursing homes, and she obtained a grant to develop specific mental health programs for elders. She was recruited to work in a new psychiatric hospital and was employed there until she was 83.

Ardis, who was born in 1912, represents the post–World War I generation of nurses and is certainly an outstanding role model that mature nurses could emulate. These characteristics include breaking the age barrier, again and again, defining for herself what aging means and not allowing someone else's definition of aging to interfere with her life goals. Her tenacious grip on productive work, which is clearly fulfilling, is reminiscent of Kahlil Gibran's poem "On Work," which begins as follows:

> You work that you may keep pace with the earth and the soul of the earth.
>
> For to be idle is to become a stranger unto the seasons, and to step out of life's procession, that marches on in majesty and proud submission towards the infinite.[12]

Ardis and each of the nurses profiled here have found that work allows them to keep step with "life's procession." Each of these nurses have made personal choices about work that not only benefited them but the nursing workforce as well and, ultimately of course, the patient. Each of these nurses defined for herself the meaning of work as well as the meaning of retirement.

WHAT IS WORK?

It is impossible to read the profiles of these mature nurses without seeing that the work experience they seek offers something intangible. Of course, the paycheck is welcome and usually necessary, but it is also important to understand what there is about work that attracts people to it. This understanding is a powerful antidote to stress and burnout at any stage in your work life, and it is even more essential to planning your mature years, whether you decide to continue working or to retire.

Before you decide to leave or replace your work, it is important to know what you are leaving behind and to understand what work means to *you* in particular. It is also important to distinguish between the job description you fulfill for your employer and the work experience you have accumulated over the span of a career, remembering that your work is eminently transportable and transformable. Only the job belongs to the employer, not your work. And it is your job and its accompanying structure that you dismantle when you retire—*not* your work or even your career. You will find more information devoted to your nursing career as an independent, self-employed, and self-directed venture, even if you are employed, in Part Two of this book.

Work meets personal as well as professional needs. It contributes to and shapes who we are as people and allows us to be part of a collective human engine of productivity, service, and progress. Work gives us a community within which to express ourselves, a place where we are known and appreciated, and a place in which to relate to others and fulfill our sense of purpose. Work gives structure, ritual, and routine to our lives.

Stress and burnout, as well as the depletion in energy that accompanies aging for some people, can interfere with our ability to remember and appreciate these essential characteristics of work as we focus on our day to day lives. Some who retire may be seeking the reduction or management of stress, not necessarily an exit from work itself. It is often this stress, in the form of untenable working conditions and employment policies, that drives the mature nurse from the workforce. And it is these conditions that employers are attempting to address with policies and programs that better accommodate the needs of mature nurses. Clearly, all nurses stand to benefit from this attention.

Our fascination with work begins early in life. As children, we imitate the work we see our parents do. We busy ourselves with the "work" of play in which we learn about ourselves and the world around us. For the many adults who find fulfillment and expression in their work, our work becomes a type of "play." This can include nurses, of course. Listen carefully to nurses who have lost the enjoyment that work can bring, and what you hear is the stress of too many patients with too few nurses to care for them along with unfair, ineffective, or even harmful workplace policies—not the work of making a difference in the lives of others, not the "play" of work so to speak. Sadly, for far too many nurses, the decision to retire may be the only way out.

Work sharpens, toughens, and strengthens us, mentally and physically, with its challenges, demands, and discipline. Remember the profile of Jacqueline Khan who "wanted work to be difficult"? Work defines who we are and becomes a source of our identity, of how we think about ourselves and how we answer the question "What do you do?" Not being able to answer this question is often the first sign that something big is missing in retirement. Work is so identified with who we are that we ask children what they want to be when they grow up. Dismantling one's work during the mature years seems unnecessary when the option for a working retirement is possible. For others, the preference is to translate their knowledge and skills into volunteer experiences.

Let's revisit how work is described by Kahlil Gibran, the 20th-century poet and mystic, in his poem "On Work":

> You work that you may keep pace with the earth and the soul of the earth.
> For to be idle is to become a stranger unto the seasons, and to step out of life's procession, that marches on in majesty and proud submission towards the infinite.
> When you work you are a flute through whose heart the whispering of the hours turns to music.
> Which of you would be a reed, dumb and silent, while all else sings together in unison?

> Always you have been told that work is a curse and labour a misfortune.
> But I say to you that when you work you fulfill a part of earth's dream, assigned to you when that dream was born,
> And in keeping yourself with labour you are in truth loving life,
> And to love life through labour is to be intimate with life's inmost secret.
> Work is love made visible.
> (Kibran, 1973)[12]

Embedded in this poem are questions on which you could reflect in order to consider the meaning work has for you. Return periodically to these questions (and others you may be asking) as you prepare for and move through this stage of your life.

- In what way does your work allow you to "keep pace with the earth"; that is, to stay current with events, people, places, ideas?
- With what would you replace your work so that you didn't "step out of life's procession"—so that you were still in step with what was meaningful to you?
- Ignoring for a moment the stress that may accompany your work, how might you describe the "music" of your work? Consider here the "song" of your work, so to speak—what it is like for you to give your gift of caring to another and to do this as part of a team "singing together in unison."
- Do you think your work is a "curse" or that your labor/work is a "misfortune"? If you've been told this by others, do you believe them? Or is it possible that the "song" of your work is hard to "sing" because of workplace practices and relationships that create stress. Perhaps this is what you want to leave behind, not necessarily the "song" itself. Alternatively you may be ready for a different "dream," a different "song," but as yet be unsure the form it will take. Or you may already know and love this "song" of your work, and leaving it behind feels impossible.
- Is your work as a nurse the fulfillment of a "part of earth's dream, assigned to you when that dream was born"? Did you "dream" or at least fulfill a goal of becoming a nurse for a reason that has been satisfying and is now difficult to leave? Perhaps instead, your dream, your goals, in becoming a nurse are not yet fulfilled and might not be in your current work. What work can you now "dream" that might still achieve this goal?
- Again for the moment disregarding the stress that may accompany your work, is there a desire to continue to "love life through [the] labour" that is nursing so as to be close to "life's inmost secret"?

- Can you imagine your work as a nurse as "love made visible"? And, just as important, in what way will your love continue to be visible—to be expressed—should you decide to leave nursing behind?

There are no right or wrong answers to these questions. There are only your very personal responses to the meaning work has for you. Your answers can help put you in touch with how to take your work into the next phase of your life and shape your retirement, whether working or not.

WHAT IS RETIREMENT?

As more and more people decide to work past age 65, the historically accepted age of retirement, defining what *retirement* means is difficult at best. Taking a closer look at how people are constructing their lives at age 65 and beyond, it appears that in these early years of the 21st century, we are retiring the 20th century idea of retirement! By the way, the idea of retirement did not exist before the 20th century; it is a relatively recent cultural phenomenon.[13]

Peter Drake, vice president for Fidelity Investments in Toronto, pondered the following about retirement: "The fact that so many boomers are planning to retire early and then keep on working raises a very interesting question. If you work in retirement, are you actually retired?"[13] No, says Marc Freedman, author of *Encore: Finding Work That Matters in the Second Half of Your Life,* the chapter from which Drake's question is taken. Freedman goes on to present the following historical summary about retirement:

> "First we stretched retirement from a brief hiatus that was supposed to cover the few remaining years between disability and death and turned it into a period lasting fifteen, twenty, twenty-five years. It became grotesque, unworkable for individuals and unsustainable for American society. More recently, we've been stretching the meaning of the word until it becomes similarly meaningless." (Freedman 2007, page 118)

In an article for Futurist.com, Glen Hiemstra identifies myths about retirement. The first is that 65 is old, the second is that those over 65 are generally not capable of useful work, and the third is those remaining in the paid labor force will, through Social Security tax contributions, pay for the benefits of retirees (*www.futurist.com/archives/future-trends/the-end-of-retirement-is-near/*).

We all know the facts about these myths. First, those who are 65 are no longer considered old and can anticipate having at least another 20 to 40 years of life ahead. Second, many people over 65 in the 21st century are primarily knowledge workers (such as nurses), not laborers as they were in the 20th century. Mental acuity, not muscle strength, is what is mostly needed to work today. And using the knowledge of mature nurses in the roles of educator, consultant, and preceptor, for example, is one retention strategy being utilized by healthcare employers, as will be discussed later in this chapter.

And that third myth about Social Security supporting retirees for decades is certainly not true by all accounts. It is common knowledge that retirees will require sources of income in addition to Social Security. This is often why mature workers stay in or return to the workforce. Heimstra notes with interest that when the Social Security system was established, the age to begin collecting benefits was set at 65 because the average life span at that time was 63. It was anticipated that few people would collect benefits for very long.

Perhaps looking at the dictionary definition of the word *retirement* will help us better understand its meaning and influence. To start with, *retirement* is derived from the French word *retirer,* which has two meanings. The first is "to withdraw to some place for the sake of seclusion," and the second is "to leave company and go to bed" (*www.etymonline.com*). A definition closer to our understanding of the idea of retirement is "removal or withdrawal from service, office or business" (*dictionary.reference.com*). Synonyms for the word *retirement* are interesting to note. They include *withdrawal, seclusion, retreat, departure, end, terminate, conclude, leave, put out,* and *go to bed.*

Most of these words do not fully describe the retirement experience people are actually having these days. They seem to imply a removal of oneself from people or situations that were once stimulating or engaging. There is implied a replacement of something life affirming with a kind of nothingness and isolation. Also implied in these words is an idleness that Gibran thought would make you "a stranger unto the seasons" and require that you "step out of life's procession" (Gibran 1973).

Since none of these definitions seems to capture what mature workers are doing or planning for, is it necessary to revise the meaning of *retirement* and perhaps to find a new term for it. If not *retirement,* then what? What are we to call this important and relatively new life stage? Ken Dychtwald, a gerontologist and author of *Age Wave: How the Most Important Trend of Our Time Will Change the Future,* votes for keeping the word *retirement* but changing its meaning. He says:

> But that's not how people are using the word now. We are discarding one model of retirement and embracing another. People see it as a period of engagement, of being involved and pursuing new dreams.

> There is a sense of self-determination.... Retirement means the end of work, but everybody's talking about wanting to work. Clearly, a new definition of retirement is emerging. (Brock 2008)[14]

On the other hand, Marc Freedman believes it is time to create a new category of thinking and a new language to recognize that we are entering fresh territory and shaping a new stage of life. He encourages the marketing of possibilities of this "second half of work" and uses the word *encore* to describe this.

In addition to *encore*, many other words are emerging in an attempt to describe these mature years of productivity, including *second act* and *third act.* And then there is a lot of wordplay replacing the word *retire* with such words as *re-wire, re-tread, re-invent, re-position, re-boot, re-vision,* etc. Votes to retire the word *retire* altogether come from the website *www.2young2retire.com,* which is designed to help people reinvent, plan for, and enjoy this next stage of life. The people behind this site think it's time for this word to go because it no longer describes the reality people are living.

ACCOMMODATING MATURE NURSES IN THE WORKPLACE

Healthcare organizations across the nation are considering the recommendations of surveys and study groups aimed at identifying what will keep mature nurses in the workforce longer or lure them back from retirement. The consensus of multiple surveys, such as the one conducted jointly by AARP and the Center for American Nurses, is that there is a need for policy change as well as work redesign, including the use of ergonomics and technology to lighten the physical workload. Frequently recommended is that mature nurses be involved as active participants in all aspects of redesign and decision making (*www.centerforamericannurses.org*).

What is important to note about the implementation of these accommodations is that they will improve the working conditions of *all* nurses, potentially retaining the pre-retiree or the soon-to-burn-out younger nurse about to flee. Joanne Disch, PhD, RN, FAAN, professor of nursing at the University of North Carolina, captures this potentially transformative news when she says:

> The accommodations that will help older nurses will in many cases improve the job for the younger set as well. For instance, since nurses have a high rate of back injuries, hospitals should bring in more equipment to help move patients. Hospitals may not be able to staff entire units with un-retired nurses but you could sure augment if we did a better job. (*www.nursezone.com*)[15]

AARP identifies five key areas that impact the recruitment and retention of the mature worker (*www.aarp.org*):

1. Ensuring meaningful work by
    - building a multigenerational workforce
    - making senior management accessible
    - conducting employee satisfaction surveys every 12–18 months
2. Improving wellness and work-life balance through
    - flexible work arrangements
    - providing elder care support
    - providing life planning courses on finances, Medicare, recreation, etc.
3. Providing training and reskilling through offerings such as
    - tuition reimbursement
    - on-site classes for computer and medical technology
    - using soon-to-retire employees to train new workers
4. Overhauling work environments and tools by
    - using mechanical lifts and lift teams
    - using ergonomically correct equipment
    - replacing faraway workstations with centralized pods
5. Improving compensation and benefits, including by
    - offering pension plans or generous matching amounts for 401(k) plans
    - providing pay scales that reflect education and experience
    - providing comprehensive health coverage

Many of these important workplace accommodations were also identified in a survey of the aging nurse conducted by the journal *Nursing Management* in partnership with the Bernard Hodes Health Group. In its findings and implications, the survey identified ANCC Magnet Hospitals as better prepared than non–Magnet Hospitals to offer the policies and programs determined as essential to retain mature nurses. They believed one possibility for this was that many of these workplace policies and practices were among the standards and criteria already specified for Magnet recognition. Their report contains an Aging Workforce Recruiter Checklist, which appears on the following page. All nurses, especially the mature nurse, could use this checklist to seek employers or who are reshaping the work environment in these respectful and inviting ways (See chapter 2 for a more about the importance of ANCC Magnet accreditation.)

Aging Workforce Recruiter Checklist

- Long-term workforce planning committees
- Succession planning
- Education/management training to fill manager pipeline
- Flexible benefits adapted to different age groups
- Ergonomics committees
- Flexible shift options of four, six, and eight hours
- Job sharing
- Patient assignments clustered to avoid extensive walking
- Lift teams and special beds/equipment to curtail injuries and strain
- Improved/special lighting for older workers (especially for computers)
- Supplies/equipment kept in central locations to avoid extensive walking
- Back care/safety training programs with annual refreshers
- Implementation of wellness programs (strength training, etc.)
- Massage or alternative therapies (acupressure, etc.)
- On-site or subsidized gym membership
- Stress-reduction training
- Use of mature nurses for nonphysical work, such as patient admission assessment
- Use of mature nurses as mentors and preceptors
- Reduction of floating for tenured employees
- Reduction of overtime requirements for tenured employees
- Mixing of age groups on projects and committees
- Intergenerational workshops
- Retiree return programs

St. Mary's Medical Center in Huntington, West Virginia, provides us with an example of a workplace accommodation program that addressed its nursing shortage and improved employee satisfaction by inviting retired nurses back to work. Following a reorientation, nurses were offered flexible schedules of fewer than 20 hours per week and fewer than 8 hours per day.

What is unique about the St. Mary's program is the freedom nurses had to create their own schedules tailored to their own needs. They had abbreviated job descriptions, including performing nursing admission assessments, changing intravenous tubing, giving pain medication, accompanying patients to off-site MRI exams, etc. Some were used in floating assignments throughout the hospital, with supervisors reaching them by portable telephones as needs emerged throughout the day.

A nurse who participated in this program wrote the letter that appears below. Her experience clearly speaks volumes about how valuable programs like this are and the potential they have to create win-win experiences for all concerned.

> To Whom It May Concern,
>
> Three years ago, at the age of 47, I found myself wondering what I was going to do now that I was facing the empty nest syndrome. I had raised three children, and the last one was ready to enter college. I received a letter in the mail describing a new program that was beginning at St. Mary's Medical Center.
>
> I was thrilled because it sounded as if it was exactly what I was looking for—a chance to get back into the field I chose 25 years ago because I loved it. But I did not want to work full-time, nor did I want to work shift work. I had not worked as a registered nurse in 25 years.
>
> St. Mary's progressive program allows me to work 20 hours a week. The best part is the program's flexibility. It allows me to pick and choose the hours and the days I want to work! It has proven to be a wonderful experience for me, and I am able to make a difference in a patient's life. I know this by the many thank-you's and hugs that I receive from them. This in turn makes me feel wonderful. I also know that I have made a difference for the nurses on each nursing unit. I have been received very well, and the appreciation that they express to me is very rewarding. Most days, I handle the nursing admission assessments of new patients. This can take up to an hour and a half, depending on the degree of the patient's current and past

medical history. I can be of such value to the emergency department and surgical recovery room when they are holding patients. I also accompany patients who need a nurse to accompany them to our off-site MRI, which enables the nurse to remain on her unit with her patients. This procedure can take up to two hours. I could go on and on about how rewarding this has been for me and how much I know that I am appreciated by the nursing units at St. Mary's Medical Center. But, trust me when I tell you, I love it!

Sincerely,
Ruth McComas

THE MULTIGENERATIONAL NURSING WORKFORCE

Every survey conducted on issues related to retaining the mature nurse recommends a focus on intergenerational relationships. Considering that four generations of nurses now comprise the nursing workforce, each with very different sets of attitudes, beliefs, work habits, and expectations, understanding how to make use of the differences *and* similarities of these four generations is essential to harmonious interpersonal relationships and team collaboration and to working in the complex and challenging conditions found in healthcare workplaces.

The nursing workforce will be age-diverse for years to come, according to Rose Sherman in her 2006 article titled "Leading a Multigenerational Nursing Workforce: Issues, Challenges and Strategies" (*nursingworld.org*). She adds:

> Although four different generations in the workforce can present leadership challenges, the diversity can also add richness and strength to the team if all staff members are valued for their contributions. In today's highly competitive healthcare market, organizations and leaders that effectively manage their age-diverse workforce will enjoy a competitive edge.... This will allow the leader to flex their leadership style, enhance quality and productivity, reduce conflict and maximize contributions of all staff.[16]

Sherman identifies the four generational cohort groups and their characteristics as follows.

The Veterans (1925–1945)

Sometimes called the GI or silent generation, this group grew up shaped by World War II and the Great Depression; economic and political uncertainty led them to be hard working, financially conservative, and cautious. They value history and look to the past for insight. They are loyal and supportive, seniority is important to them, and they possess disciplined work habits.

The Baby Boomers (1946–1964)

This generation grew up in a healthy postwar economy when individualism and creativity were encouraged. Often described as egocentric, they spent their lives rewriting rules. The largest cohort in the workforce, they have a strong work ethic, and work defines their self-worth; they occupy many leadership positions. Work accommodation efforts are targeted at this group as they prepare to retire.

Generation X (1963–1980)

Many in this generation were raised in single-parent, latchkey homes as divorce rates increased. This was the first generation with both parents commonly in the workforce and the first generation exposed to massive layoffs, leading them to value self-reliance and work-life balance. Technological advances have been an important part of their lives.

The Millennial Generation (1980–2000)

Members of this generation grew up in a time when violence, terrorism, and drugs became realities of life. They are the global generation, accepting of multiculturalism. Technology and instant communication have always been part of their lives.

Each of these generations has much to teach the other, as the profiles of Sam and Ida illustrate in chapter 4. They mentored one another in their respective areas of expertise. Ida, a mature nurse, benefited from Sam's technology and computer abilities, while Sam, a new graduate, was able to learn nursing skills and competencies under Ida's expert tutelage and reassuring presence. It is clear that multigenerational relationships are an important part of the work environment, and unless policies and programs support effective communication and relationships among these four cohorts, other work accommodation efforts will not be enough to ensure the retention of nurses, especially mature nurses.

THE DECISION TO RETIRE

Planning your career has always been important. Planning this stage of your life is just as essential. Self-exploration has never been more important. Because you are likely to be planning for approximately one-third of your life, this planning will need to be ongoing as your needs, desires, and circumstances change. How you define work and what it means to you will clearly influence how much work, if any, you want in your life during these mature years. Also, remember that there are many ways to design retirement, including the continuation of an active work life as discussed earlier. The black-and-white thinking of retirement versus work is being replaced with many shades of gray, creating at least the following kinds of "working retirement" experiences:

- Full-time work
- Part-time work
- Negotiating for shifts as short as two hours
- Working in a different industry
- Becoming an entrepreneur or consultant
- Retiring and then unretiring
- Using transferable skills or developing new skills as a volunteer

To determine what work-retirement configuration works best for you, consider using a holistic approach, which could include physical, mental, emotional, financial, and spiritual preparation. Create questions that take each of these dimensions into consideration, such as these:

- What does retirement mean to me? What exactly will I be doing? What do I see occupying my time in the years to come?
- What does work mean to me? What does it give me that I would miss and how, if at all, does it fit into this next stage of my life?
- Do I want to keep working but need to define work differently? How?
- Do I want to work but no longer as a nurse?
- What do I want to do with the portion of nursing's "brain trust" that belongs to me? Cherish it privately? Find a way to share it and pass it along?
- Do I want to use my nursing skills and experience in another way? As a volunteer? In another field?
- What are my transferable skills and experience?
- How much time do I want work to occupy in my life as I grow older?
- How would I use my time if not working? Travel? Hobbies? Grandchildren?
- Should I retire completely? If so, to what situation and activities will I retire?

- Should I semiretire, working as a nurse but differently, with fewer hours perhaps?
- Am I financially prepared for retirement? If not yet, when? How can I get there?
- Are there health issues or physical limitations to consider?
- Are there other people to consider?

It is important to recognize that there is no right or wrong answer to these questions, only *your* answers. And, just as important is to allow different answers to emerge as time passes and circumstances change in planned and unplanned ways.

Key to your decision making is keeping track of emerging employment opportunities for the mature nurse. Despite some of the physical demands placed on nurses by their work, it is important to remember that nurses are knowledge workers and age is not a barrier to working in this way. In fact, is likely to be a plus. Aware of this, healthcare employers are creating work options heretofore unheard of that might suit your needs. Or if none exists yet in your area, consider talking to your employer and suggesting alterations in your work assignments like those in the examples below (*www.nurseweek.com/news/Features/04-09/RetiredRNs_print.html*):[17]

- The ReturN program at The Rogue Valley Medical Center in Medford, Oregon, offers retired nurses their choice of work schedules and assignments. Many mature nurses opt to work two- to four-hour shifts during times of peak activity, some as direct care nurses and others as trainers for new equipment. Nurses are paid an hourly rate without benefits except for pharmacy discounts.
- The ValleyCare Health System in Livermore, California, has a Nursing Alumni Guild, whose members are retired nurses and raise money to buy medical equipment for the hospital. They are also used as mentors for nursing students and have opportunities to keep current with nursing and healthcare developments though classes the hospital offers.
- The Poudre Valley Health System in Fort Collins, Colorado, introduced a program called REACH (Re-entering Acute Care Hospitals) aimed at encouraging retired nurses to return to work by providing reorientation classes that met their particular needs rather than including them in the regular new employee orientation, where they might have felt uncomfortable.

Additional job options for mature nurses might include the following:

- Working as a home care nurse in shifts of four or more hours visiting continuous-care patients close to your home
- Working as a substitute school nurse on an as-needed basis
- Working for agencies that employ nurses to give influenza immunizations at local clinics for shifts as short as two hours on days of your choice
- Becoming a travel nurse and combining your itch to travel with your desire to continue working. This might be ideal for the mature nurse who has adult children or grandchildren in another part of the country.
- Considering telenursing, where you interact with patients on the phone. You might be assessing physical status, providing health counseling, participating in research protocols, etc.

THRIVING AS A MATURE NURSE

Make Sure Your Voice Is Heard: Be Part of the Dialogue

Your opinions count heavily here. Healthcare organizations are gearing up to develop strategies to recruit and retain you in the workforce. Make sure they know what you need to make that happen, such as flexible hours and so on. Be sure to maintain your professionalism by being realistic about your requests; look for win-win options that benefit you *and* the organization. Track the discussion about this important issue any way you can. Go to conferences, read nursing journals and newsletters, and, of course, get online and "hear" what others are saying and doing. Go to the Academy of Medical Surgical Nurses website (*www.medsurgnurse.org*) to find out about its mentoring program called Nurses Nurturing Nurses, or N3 for short.

Self-Care Really Counts Now!

This is especially true for physical self-care. Whatever you were able to get away with when you were younger may be less possible now. If you want to remain a contributing member of the nursing community as well as the *human* community, take your self-care seriously. This means healthy eating, adequate exercise, and sufficient rest among other things.. Refer to chapter 15 for a further discussion on self-care or to any other resource that will motivate you to take charge of this essential part of your life.

Reassess Your Nursing Skills and Competencies

Determine how you want to continue using your skills. Watch for new options that healthcare organizations are beginning to offer mature nurses and find a match between what they are offering and your reassessed skills and competencies. For example, if you are a critical care nurse who no longer desires to provide direct patient care, watch for mentoring, precepting, or teaching opportunities that do not require you to have your own patient care assignment.

Choose If and How You Want to Continue Working

Accurately assess your physical, mental, emotional, spiritual, and personal stamina. Be realistic about what you can and cannot do. Your journey as a nurse may not be over yet. You may want to consider allowing it to continue longer for the benefit of other nurses who will follow in your footsteps and for those for whom they will care. After all, isn't the experience of making a difference a primary reason you became a nurse to begin with?

If You Choose Not to Continue Working

Celebrate your nursing achievements and accomplishments. Moving on to other experiences following a nursing career is just as important a decision as continuing to work, as long as it is a conscious choice made after deliberating and reflecting on your options.

Keep Current

Stay informed about current clinical and professional issues and about the healthcare field in general. The best way to stay current is to use several websites and/or listservs, especially those of the American Nurses Association (*nursingworld.org*) or your state nurses association. Refer to chapter 4 or the Resources section at the end of this book for more information.

Provide Wisdom, Not Warnings

In your mentoring and preceptor relationships, be sure you are sharing what's right and great about nursing, how far we've come, and where we still need to go. Share the lessons learned and the progress made. There is reason for optimism, even when the challenges are great. If you have trouble believing this—if you are of the opinion that "things never change"—reconsider whether mentoring is the right choice for you. This is not a time for doom-and-gloom thinking. If you must tell your war stories, tell them with a balanced perspective of then versus now and consider including a healthy dose of optimism and perhaps humor.

Yours Is the Past, the Present, and the Future

Just as new graduates straddle the two worlds between school and work, so do mature nurses straddle the worlds between two centuries, the 20th and the 21st, the time between old and new, between past and present. For those of you who choose to stay on in nursing, you have an opportunity to influence the world of nursing yet to be—the future. Yours is an opportunity to contribute in ways you might not have imagined five or ten years ago.

YOUR ROAD AHEAD

There are many paths to take as a mature nurse, and as Robert Frost taught us, the path you choose can "make all the difference!"

The Road Not Taken

Two roads diverged in a yellow wood,
And sorry I could not travel both
And be one traveler, long I stood
And looked down one as far as I could
To where it bent in the undergrowth;

Then took the other, as just as fair
And having perhaps the better claim,
Because it was grassy and wanted wear;
Though as for that the passing there
Had worn them really about the same,

And both that morning equally lay
In leaves no step had trodden black,
Oh, I kept the first for another day!
Yet knowing how way leads on to way,
I doubted if I should ever come back.

I shall be telling this with a sigh
Somewhere ages and ages hence:
Two roads diverged in a wood, and I—
I took the one less traveled by,
And that has made all the difference.

—Robert Frost[18]

CHAPTER 7

Men: The Changing Face of Nursing

> Today men are resuming their historical role as caring, nurturing nurses, just as some women are resuming their roles as physicians. After a century as a predominantly female profession, nursing is changing again. It will be interesting to see what happens in the next century.
>
> —Men in American Nursing History, *Bruce Wilson, PhD, RN (www.geocities.com/~brucewilson/)*[2]

According to the most recent National Sample Survey of Registered Nurses in 2008, 6.6 percent of the American RN workforce was male.[1] Although this number was up from 5.8 percent in the previous survey in 2004, in this age of increasing tolerance for ethnic diversity and an ever-growing awareness of the damaging effect of gender barriers, the fact that nursing is still a profession comprised of 93 percent women should raise a red flag of concern. This is especially true if the profession's current difficulty attracting people (women and men alike) is contributing to a risk of not meeting the healthcare needs of American society. The National Advisory Council on Nursing Education and Practice warns that if nursing, which represents the largest healthcare profession, is to address the unique needs of this country's growing minority populations, it is vital that they attract more men and minorities.[3]

The shortage of nurses is a crisis and, like all crises, offers opportunities for something new and different to happen, including the possibility of something better. Increasing the presence of men in a profession long dominated by women may well represent something better.

Attracting more men into nursing is certainly not the only answer to the nursing shortage or to ensuring America's healthcare needs. And, clearly, the 94 percent female professionals in nursing are not waiting for, nor do they need to be "rescued" from, their current difficulties by men. However, increasing the diversity, gender included, of any group of people has been shown to have positive effects on its culture, once barriers to diversity are identified and eliminated. There is every reason to believe this to be true for the culture of nursing as well. Interestingly, while nursing has made some inroads to increasing its cultural diversity, the same cannot be said of its gender mix.

THE GLASS GATE?

Some of what is experienced by men today seeking to become nurses or already working as nurses is reminiscent of what women experienced, and are still experiencing, as they enter male-dominated professions in healthcare, especially when they aim high and find themselves blocked by the so-called "glass ceiling." If women experience a "glass ceiling," do men entering nursing experience a "glass gate?" Why does the gate exist? What experiences do men have trying to get through it? What successful strategies for opening this gate are individuals, institutions, and organizations using? Who are the men that have succeeded in getting to the other side? How will the nursing profession and the healthcare industry benefit from the presence of more men?

The sections that follow begin to address these questions and ask others. You are invited to add your own answers to these questions, to think of additional questions, and to ask these questions among your professional and personal networks to increase awareness and generate solutions that can open wide the "glass gate."

WHY THE GLASS GATE EXISTS

In an article titled "Men and Women in Nursing" in the April 28, 2008, issue of *Advance for Nurses*, Gail O. Guteri asks, "History shows men were a force in nursing before the 1860s; what caused them to become a minority in the profession?" She attempts to answer this question in an interview with Russell Eugene Tranbarger, EdD, RN, FAAN, who suggests that Florence Nightingale herself may have started this trend with her writings and development of modern nursing. He notes that "her book didn't say men can't be nurses, but she never refers to men." Because of the poor nursing she observed from male nurses in the Crimean war, and in an attempt to create a profession for women outside the home, "she had to prove that men weren't capable of doing nursing, because at that time, men were very present in nursing." He goes on to say that he and other men in the profession "bear no ill will" toward Nightingale and notes, "It wasn't for evil purposes, but it was clearly her intent to drive us out. It was the only way [she] could achieve her goal."[4]

Whatever its origins, clearly the glass gate continues to exist. In its December 2001 *Issues Bulletin*, the American Association of Colleges of Nursing (*www.aacn.nche.edu*) identified the following reasons men and minority group members do not pursue nursing:

- Role stereotypes
- Economic barriers
- Few mentors
- Gender biases
- Lack of direction from early authority figures
- Misunderstanding about the practice of nursing
- Increased opportunities in other fields[5]

Michael Williams, RN, MSN, CCRN, was the first male president of the American Association of Critical Care Nurses. In the August 2001 issue of *AACN News* (www.*aacn.org*), his "President's Notes: A Journey of Rediscovery—So How Does It Feel to You?" identified the following "host of challenges" facing men who choose nursing:

- Invisibility
- Negative stereotypes
- Few male faculty members in nursing schools
- Male students socialized to downplay their gender
- Little opportunity to work and communicate with other men in nursing
- Misperceptions about their competence and qualifications for promotion
- Differences in how each gender communicates
- Perceptions that physicians automatically respect men in nursing more than women
- Perhaps the most devaluing of all, the perception that a man cannot be caring and compassionate enough to be a nurse[6]

Some of these challenges are echoed by Chad E. O'Lynn, PhD, RN, coeditor of the book *Men in Nursing: History, Challenges, and Opportunities* (O'Lynn &

Tranbarger 2007). He identifies a gendered construction of nursing as being a barrier to men considering entering the profession. Other gender-based barriers, such as the feminine paradigm in nursing education, the lack of male role models and isolation, the use of gender-biased language, differential treatment, different styles of communication, and issues of touch and caring, are all possible causes for stress among male nursing students and may lead to higher attrition and failure rates.[7]

ROLE STEREOTYPES AND GENDER BIASES

The leaders of the National Student Nurses Association (NSNA) recognize that getting men interested in nursing careers requires male as well as female role models. In a question-and-answer column called "Breakthrough to Nursing" (*Imprint* 2002), Ashleigh Williams and Nikki Battle encourage "those participating in 'Breakthrough to Nursing' projects, particularly in elementary schools, to ensure that those representing nursing are a diverse group that include men."[8]

The idea that women become nurses and men become physicians is so deeply entrenched in the American psyche that as recently as July 2002, an article in a nursing publication that discussed nurse-physician relationships showed a drawing of a man in a white coat, pounding his fist in anger to make a point to a woman in casual professional dress with her arms folded across her chest. There was no caption under the picture, leaving it to the reader to decide who was the nurse and who was the physician. This was not difficult, since throughout, the article used feminine pronoun *she* when referring to the nurse and the masculine pronoun *he* when referring to the physician. Would it have been illuminating or confusing if in the article, *she* referred to the physician and *he* to the nurse? In what ways might nursing and the media be responsible for reinforcing the myths and stereotypes that become glass gates?

Among today's 6 percent of nurses who are men, there are some impressive role models. Michael Desjardins, RN, the first male president of the National Student Nurses' Association, is one of them. He represents someone who succeeded in getting through the gate and is now in a position to influence how others might do so as well. In an article called "Looking for a Few Good Men" by Debra Williams in the spring 2002 issue of *Minority Nurse* (*minoritynurse.com*), Desjardins critiques a popular movie, a comedy called *Meet the Parents*, in which the actor Ben Stiller is seeking to marry a woman whose parents do not approve of him for many reasons, most particularly because he is a male nurse, the basis of many jokes throughout the movie. In this article, Desjardins discusses how he knows too well that these fictional jokes are the reality for men who have chosen nursing as a career. He states, "After all of the chaos [Stiller's character causes], the one thing the father can't forgive is that he is a male nurse. I don't see that as funny." Williams notes, "Desjardins confronts stereotypes about male nurses practically every day. People act surprised when they learn his occupation. Friends have told him to wear his wedding ring to work so people won't assume he's gay. Even though he's only been an RN for a year, [he] is already concerned about the effects his gender may have on his career path."[9]

THE PUBLIC'S IMAGE OF NURSES

What the public thinks of the nurse in terms of appearance, perceived functions, prestige and what they hear nurses say (or don't hear, as the case may be) ultimately determine the perceived value of nursing as a career choice. That nursing is not seen as prestigious a career choice as medicine indicates two problems. The first is that caregiving and nurturing, central (though certainly not the only) functions of professional nursing, are not seen as important or essential. The second problem involves the difficulty in recruiting people, men or women, to a profession that is devalued and misunderstood.

This devalued image of the nurse results from long-held and unattractive stereotypes as well as a misunderstanding of what nurses actually do. It is often hard for the public to know how to identify a nurse among other healthcare personnel. In "The Image of Nursing: Past, Present and Future" in the February/March 2002 issue of *Imprint* (*www.nsna.org*), Michael Evans, at that time a member of the board of directors of NSNA and editor of *Imprint*, its official publication, wrote that there is a disconnect on the part of the public about nurses. One problem is the representation of the nurse in the media, which shows "her" in a white uniform and cap, both of which were discarded by nurses in the late '70s and early '80s in favor of the more relaxed look of colorful scrubs. While the scrubs are the preferred garb today, they can create confusion in determining who the professional nurse caregiver is among the myriad of healthcare personnel who all dress alike.[10]

Compounding the problem of the nurse's image is that the voice of the nurse is strikingly absent from the media as an expert spokesperson. "The Woodhull Study on Nursing and the Media," an oft-quoted research project conducted in 1997 by Sigma Theta Tau International (*www.nursingsociety.org*), published key findings, three of which are described below.

1. On average, nurses were cited only 3 percent of the time in hundreds of health-related articles culled from 16 major news publications.
2. In seven newspapers surveyed, nurses and nursing were referenced in only 4 percent of the healthcare articles examined. The few references to nurses or nursing were mostly in passing.
3. Articles examined during the study referred to both physicians and healthcare academics as doctors. No example was found where a nurse with a doctorate was referred to as doctor.[11]

The idea that what nurses do is dictated by and supervised by physicians is inaccurate but firmly believed and widely pervasive. Nor is nursing usually a stepping-stone to becoming a physician, as so many people think. Nursing and medicine are collaborative professions, often sharing responsibility for the same patients, but with a different, albeit overlapping, focus. Nurses are experts in wellness and coping, rather than extensions of the medical profession.

The widely used phrase *doctor's orders* refers to medical regimens that are prescribed for a patient and expected to be executed by the nurse, based on the nurse's professional judgment. Nurses who blindly carry out medical regimens without regard for how the status of the patient may indicate otherwise or the appropriateness of the order are failing in their responsibility to protect the patient from harm. Such lack of action regarding professional nursing judgment can result in discipline or revocation of one's license. The interdependence and thoughtful collaboration of the professions of nursing and medicine is usually misunderstood by the public.

EXPERIENCES OF MEN IN NURSING

Who are the men who make it through the glass gate? In 2004, the Bernard Hodes Group, a marketing research firm, in collaboration with the California Institute for Nursing & Health Care and Coalition for Nursing Careers in California and in consultation with the American Assembly for Men in Nursing, surveyed 498 men across the country who were staff nurses, clinical managers, and educators. They found that the top reason for entering nursing was the desire to help people, followed by nursing being a growth profession with many career paths, the desire to have a stable career, and a variety of geographical choices. Many of these men entered nursing as a second career rather than directly after high school, often after the military or other health careers. They often chose employment in trauma, critical care, and other areas that offer autonomy and technological challenges, and they are committed to their careers despite multiple challenges they face related to working in a largely female field, such as stereotypes, lack of role models, and feelings of isolation.[12]

Following are some descriptions of men who tell what it is like for them to be a nurse. Listen to the good, the bad, and the hopeful experiences of these men. In these passages, you will hear examples of the barriers and obstacles described in the previous pages. Listen also for what these men have done to overcome what they were facing, as well as what still awaits to be done. Michael Williams, continuing in "President's Notes: A Journey of Rediscovery—So How Does It Feel to You?" notes that "nursing continues to be a profession that allows situations to occur, like these from my own experience:

- "'Don't let yourself be promoted too soon,' I was advised. 'Hospitals have a habit of promoting men who aren't qualified.' Even today I'm haunted by the possibility that some of my promotions have been because of my gender, not my competence.
- "A week before I accepted a faculty position, the men's restroom became a storage room. 'There are no men in nursing,' I was told.
- "The lone male student in a class struggled to develop his physical assessment skills because he couldn't practice on female classmates, though they could practice on him.
- "Recently, when a group of us were introduced as 'the critical care nurse group,' the introducer failed to acknowledge me, because he didn't see me as a nurse."

Williams goes on to say, "Admittedly, these unfortunate examples do not tell the entire story. Fortunately, I also know about experiences like these:

- "The clinical instructor contacted the student to ask him, 'Do you have any questions or concerns that I could help you clarify before you start your women's health rotation?'
- "'I need a nurse to assist me,' the obstetrician told the delivery room nurse manager, who responded, 'Let me introduce you to your patient's nurse; he is right here.'
- "'Your [female] classmates seem to have a problem that my nurse is a man,' the 19-year-old woman said to the male student. 'I don't see anything unusual about a man being a nurse, do you?'
- "When the new graduate was asked why she chose nursing as a career, she replied, 'Because my father is a nurse.'"

Four nurses featured in an article by Mildred Culp in the May 13, 2008, *New York Daily News* titled "Stereotypes Down for Male Nurses" are emblematic of men entering nursing as a second career.

William Donoghue, psychiatric nurse, 60, went into nursing a few years after returning from Vietnam. Helped by the GI Bill, he dropped bartending and enrolled in a hospital school of nursing. He actually took a pay cut from his former job, but he and his wife wanted to have children so he needed a job with benefits and stability. Today, he earns $95,000 working with kids at a medical center in the Bronx and knows he is making a difference. "There are few careers that give you that sense of satisfaction," he said.

James Angehr, home healthcare nurse, 45, didn't leave his 16-year career as a computer systems analyst for a large corporation for the money—he did it for a better lifestyle. He found the heavy commute, high stress, and deadlines of his former job taxing. He was willing to go down in salary and work more with people, but he didn't know about nursing until a pal working as a nurse suggested it. He enrolled in an accelerated nursing program and within two years was able to trade three hours of commuting for a job in his own neighborhood with a visiting nurse service, earning a bit more than $70,000 a year.

Jorge Prada, nursing student, 38, originally worked as a bank teller in his native Venezuela. When he immigrated to the United States, he worked as a personal trainer and waiter while trying to figure out a long-term career plan. He met a nurse in 2004 who "told me that I fit the profile." He is now a junior in nursing school and said he can't wait to get started. "I love caring for people and helping others," he said.

Peter Muncar, 43, worked as a doctor in his native Yugoslavia. He left for New York when his country was moving toward war in 1990. He now works as a home care nurse, working with about 130 elderly clients. He assesses their medical and social needs, including those of the patient's family, and then helps them to tap into the professionals they need. Although trained as a doctor in Romania, he's content working as a nurse and earning a salary of around $65,000. "You don't get rich, but you are in the middle class," he says.[13]

Don Paradise was a nursing student at Mount Saint Mary's College in Newburgh, New York, when he was featured in a June 24, 2002, article in *Advance for Nurses* called "Paradise Lost No More" by Alan Snel (*nursing.advanceweb.com*). In the article, Paradise is described as "emblematic of the new face of nurses." He is a 25-year-old, 6-foot 6-inch who played for his college's basketball team and one day wants to be an emergency flight nurse. While completing his studies, he was working in a Level II trauma center, excited about the fast-paced action and how he was able to apply the assessment skills he was learning in school. Snel describes that Paradise

> joked about how banter among female nurses dies down when he enters a room. He theorized that men might not enter nursing because they look at nursing as a feminine role.... "There's no feminine side to nursing.... I want to see men be completely comfortable in this role and not feel scrutinized."

The article ends with the following words of advice from Paradise: "You should do stuff to be happy. I don't think gender should have anything to do with it. You have to want to care for people."[14]

In "Still Not Much of a Guy Thing" in *Hopkins Nurse* (a publication of the Johns Hopkins Hospital), Anne Bennett Swingle profiles a number of men whose self-reported invigorating experiences being a nurse represent a turning tide.

Tom Galloway, a veteran emergency medicine nurse, says that, "Nearly one quarter of all RNs in emergency medicine are men, and that's enough to turn the traditional equations upside down." According to Swingle, "Galloway recalls shifts in the ER when all the doctors were women and all the nurses were men."

The first job for Kevin McDonald, a new BSN graduate, was in the cardiac surgical ICU. "It's quite a trip," McDonald says, looking back on all he learned. "The acuity of the patients is high; you really have to have the stomach for it." He goes on to say, "I have friends who make more money, but when I compare my average day to theirs, mine is more challenging and exciting. And when I describe the sort of things I do every day, they are awestruck."

Chris Boyle, who has been a psychiatric nurse for 15 years, has been able to find all the variety and satisfaction he's ever needed without ever leaving the floor. "At every point, whenever I wanted something new, an opportunity would always open up." This included participating in opening up a day hospital where he is now the nurse manager, supervising a staff of 45 RNs and other caregivers.

A longtime psychiatric nurse, Gary Dunn leads a monthly support group for male students at the Hopkins School of Nursing. Dunn started the group when he became aware that the students missed having a peer group and role models. A common problem with which they often struggle is that their family and friends see nursing as a stepping-stone to becoming a physician.[15]

Despite representing a minority of the nursing profession, each of the men profiled here have found their way through the "glass gate" where they model gender-neutral behavior, resist being stereotyped, and point the way to nursing's future.

NURSING'S FUTURE AND NURSING'S ROOTS

In nursing, we are living in an era between a profession dominated by women and one that is gender-neutral, a time that foretells that the term *male nurse* will fade from use, replaced by the word *nurse* to describe both men and women who perform that role. In many ways, this change to gender neutrality will reconnect nursing with its ancient and not-so-distant historical roots, well documented at the award-winning website "Men in American Nursing History" by Bruce Wilson, PhD, RN (*www.geocities.com/~brucewilson/*). Read what Wilson has to say and recognize how the sure-to-be increase of men in nursing is about to circle us back to our roots:

> Since the earliest times, men and women have been engaged in the practices we today call nursing. These individuals combined biological, nutritional, social, aesthetic, and spiritual support. While they have been called medicine men or witch doctors, these terms indicate a lack of understanding of the significance of their contribution, and that the healer may have been either gender.
>
> The first nursing school in the world was started in India in about 250 BC. Only men were considered "pure" enough to become nurses. In the New Testament, the Good Samaritan paid the innkeeper to provide care for an injured man. No one thought it odd that a man should be paid to provide nursing care.
>
> In every plague that swept Europe, men risked their lives to provide nursing care. A group of men, the Parabolani, in 300 AD started a hospital and provided nursing care during the black plague epidemic.
>
> Seventy years before the Pilgrims landed on Plymouth Rock, Fray (Friar) Juan de Mena was shipwrecked off the south Texas coast. He is the first identified nurse in what was to become the United States.
>
> During the Civil War, both sides had military men serving as nurses although we only hear about the Union volunteers, who were predominately female. The Confederate Army identified thirty men per regiment to care for the wounded. Men, including the poet, Walt Whitman, served as volunteers in the Union Army.

OPENING THE GLASS GATE: HOW TO ATTRACT MEN INTO THE NURSING PROFESSION

The conditions, myths, and stereotypes that inhibited free access to and equal opportunity within the nursing profession for men and women alike in the 20th century cannot and must not continue into the 21st century. Recognizing that barriers must be identified and removed, many individuals, organizations, and institutions are developing strategies for recruiting and retaining male nurses. Everyone within the healthcare industry, most especially nurses, needs to take responsibility for the part they play in constructing, maintaining, and ultimately eliminating the glass gate.

Organizations

Nurses for a Healthier Tomorrow is a coalition of 43 nursing and healthcare organizations (*nursesource.org*) working together to launch an extensive communications and advertising campaign, which it describes as a grassroots effort aimed at increasing the attractiveness of nursing as a profession. Its print advertisements and public service announcements present an image of nursing as a career for everyone, inclusive of all minorities, including men, in which professionalism, teamwork, and leadership are key.

Johnson & Johnson, the world's most comprehensive manufacturer of health care products, launched "The Campaign for Nursing's Future," a multiyear, national initiative to celebrate nurses and their contributions, as well as to recruit them and the faculty to train them. This highly acclaimed effort was developed in collaboration with nursing organizations, schools, hospitals, and other healthcare groups and will be sustained with the assistance of an advisory group of nursing leaders. It features men prominently in print and television ads titled "Because I'm a Nurse" and "Dare to Care." The website (*discovernursing.com*) features career information and dozens of profiles of male and female RNs and nursing students.

Broadening diversity among healthcare workers by including men as well as other underutilized personnel sources is among the recommendations of the American Hospital Association (AHA) for solving the crisis of the nursing shortage, as outlined in the AHA Commission on Workforce for Hospitals and Health Systems' *In Our Hands: How Hospital Leaders Can Build a Thriving Workforce* (*www.aha.org*) The Commission identified five keys to solving its workforce shortages and has charged its membership with implementing them. One of these five keys is to broaden the base of its workers by:

- aggressively developing a more diverse workforce pool;
- creating attraction strategies for each generational cohort;
- pursuing people from the full range of potential sources; and
- communicating a positive, satisfying, and inspiring image of healthcare careers.[17]

The American Assembly for Men in Nursing (AAMN) is a national forum for "nurses as a group to meet, discuss, and influence factors which affect men as nurses." It has the following objectives:

- Encourage men to become nurses and join with all nurses in humanizing healthcare.
- Encourage nurses who are men to grow professionally and demonstrate contributions made by men in nursing.
- Encourage all members to participate fully in the nursing profession and its organizations.

AAMN sponsors annual conferences, produces a quarterly newsletter, and offers annual awards for organizations and individuals who are supportive of men in nursing.[19] In 2007, AAMN partnered with Johnson and Johnson's Campaign for Nursing's Future to offer a new scholarship program for male students pursuing professional nursing education programs. Twenty awardees from 15 different states were the 2007 winners.[20]

Colleges and Schools of Nursing

In its *Issue Bulletin* "Effective Strategies for Increasing Diversity in Nursing Programs," the American Association of Colleges in Nursing (*www.aacn.nche.edu*) examines some of the techniques that are working to recruit men and minorities that can be duplicated across the country:

- The University of Texas Health Science Center at Houston convened a forum of male nurses to find out what drew them to the profession. Some of the advice they gave, as described by Patricia Stark, DSN, RN, FAAN, dean of the School of Nursing, was to "play up the macho aspects of nursing, that is, emergency care and trauma, to advertise for students in the sports pages, and play up the longhorn symbol of UT. And, they told us to go back and proof our recruitment brochures and take out any flowery, feminine language." This resulted in the percentage of male students jumping to an impressive 29 percent of the student population.

- Part of a gift of $1.2 million given to the University of Maryland by Gilden Integrated, a Baltimore-based public relations firm, financed a comprehensive marketing campaign to focus on the many career opportunities in nursing. An ethnically diverse mix of men and women was featured, which is credited, in part, for a 37 percent increase in applications in the fall of 2001.
- Nancy Mills, PhD, RN, dean at the University of Missouri–Kansas City School of Nursing, used a federal grant to launch a three-year project to increase enrollment, specifically targeting men and minority groups and resulting in a class composed of 15 percent men.
- Mount Carmel College of Nursing has established the Learning Trails program, which provides one-on-one attention and mentoring to assist men throughout their college experience. This program has helped the school achieve retention and graduation rates that exceed the national average.
- In the 2001–2002 academic year, the efforts of the College of Nursing at the University of Nebraska Medical Center to reach out to men and minorities were rewarded by an increase in the applications and admissions of male students to 54 percent and 77 percent respectively. Among the strategies used was updating the marketing materials to include images and colors that were "male-friendly."

Retaining male nursing students is equally crucial to opening the glass gate. Chad O'Lynn, cited in another article by Debra Williams in the Winter 2006 issue of *Minority Nurse* titled "Recruiting Men into Nursing School" (*minoritynurse.com*), suggested the following to make nursing programs male-friendly: using gender-neutral language and gender-neutral images, ensuring that male and female students have the same learning experiences, acknowledging and addressing male concerns such as the appropriate use of touch, understanding that male students may communicate differently than female students, and observing for additional stress in male students and offering support.[21]

Here are two examples of "male-friendly" learning environments:

1. John Leighty, in an article titled "It's a Guy Thing" in the Fall 2007 issue of *Future Nurse,* reports on an initiative at the University of Pennsylvania called MAN-UP, an acronym for Male Association of Nursing at the University of Pennsylvania. MAN-UP has become an award-winning model for activities to attract men to nursing and to provide a forum on men's issues and concerns. As faculty advisor Christopher Lance

Coleman, RN, MS, MPH, APRN-BC, states, "We have never had a safe place for male nursing students to come together and talk about what it is like to be a nurse and a minority in nursing.... We didn't want to sit around weeping about challenges, but be proactive." The group also provides a forum to discuss male health issues, which are often "put on the back burner" in nursing classrooms. The MAN-UP model is now being replicated at other nearby universities.[22]

2. In the January 2008 issue of *Interaction* (the official publication of the AAMN), Chad O'Lynn, PhD, RN, describes a collaborative initiative between Monterey Peninsula College and the local community hospital started when an especially high attrition rate among male nursing students was discovered. This was of concern to the hospital because male graduates tended to work full-time, whereas female graduates worked at 80 percent or less time. Hospital staff, male alums, current male students, and faculty worked together to explore possible issues for male students and to strategize how to reduce male student attrition. Recommendations included increasing the visibility of men in nursing, establishing a men-only study group, and implementing a monthly "Men in Nursing" discussion group with the goal of reducing possible feelings of isolation and to "provide a safe setting for male students to share concerns they might have that interfere with their academic success, and obtain guidance from other men who understood their situations." The college received a grant from the Regional Health Occupations Resource Center, one of the first of its kind with a specific purpose to recruit and retain men in a nursing academic program.[23]

Doing Your Part to Open the Glass Gate

Described in the passage that follows are recruitment strategies suggested by Michael Williams. Listen to his voice. Then select at least one idea and do it! Encourage others to do so as well! Spread the word! Be proactive! Participate in eliminating the glass gate!

Michael Williams's Strategies for Recruitment

So, how will we overcome these challenges? Certainly not alone. We will need the understanding of not only our professional colleagues, but also others who are influential in changing traditional thinking. I say:

To all nurses: Speak with young people and community organizations about health careers. Socialize them to think of nursing as a career for women and men alike.

To men who are nurses: Make mentoring an essential ingredient of your professional work. If you're experienced, include men among your mentees. If you're a novice, include men among your mentors. Consider participating in career days at middle and high schools, as well as community youth groups. Make yourself visible to overcome invisibility!

To women who are nurses: Work with men in nursing to model effective communication across genders. Give us directions, even when we may forget to ask for them! Don't relegate them to [lifting] the obese patients because they have more strength. And don't assume nursing salaries will go up simply because there are more men in the profession. It's the work that matters, not the gender of the provider!

To parents and guidance counselors: When a boy who is caring, compassionate, intelligent, and adept in science is considering a health-related career, be sure that nursing is among the very real possibilities they consider.

To those developing solutions to the nursing shortage: Include men in promotional materials and develop recruitment initiatives aimed at men.

To outplacement consultants: Highlight nursing as a profession for both men and women.

To deans of nursing: Strive for greater gender diversity within the faculty. Highlight nursing faculty who are men, encouraging them to include male students among their mentees.

To managers: Instead of questioning the qualifications of male nurses who are promoted and anticipating their mistakes, encourage them. Coach them and mold them to be great leaders. Stop speculating that men are promoted only because they are men. Instead, assume that these men are expert and caring clinicians.

To philanthropists: Support nursing scholarship programs for under-represented groups that include men among them.

And to patients and families: Whenever you encounter a health professional whose role is unknown, ask the person, "Are you a nurse?"

As our professional journey continues, I foresee a place and time when the media reports about redistribution of gender demographics within traditional men's professions will be accompanied by articles that feature the growing redistribution of gender demographics within nursing as a traditional women's profession.

So, how does it feel? Sometimes different, other times normal, but mostly, my journey with you, it feels good!

This is how I see it. How about you?

THE OTHER SIDE OF THE GLASS GATE

Just as women changed and are changing the face of medicine, so will men (and other minorities) change the face of nursing, with benefits for nurses, physicians, and ultimately the patients they care for. Because men and women are different, the presence of more men is quite likely to influence nursing's relationship styles and communication patterns, particularly with physicians, which historically have been troubled and problematic.

That men and women are different is captured in the expression "Men are from Mars and women are from Venus," the title of a bestselling book that describes how the styles of relating, patterns of communicating, attributes, and viewpoints of each gender naturally create differences and how, despite them, both men and women benefit and learn from one another.

Alternatively, when men or women are the dominant gender in a group, the extremes of stereotypical feminine and masculine attributes can potentially develop. A developmental goal of each individual, male or female, is to work toward wholeness, one characteristic of which is the capacity to embrace and express both the masculine and feminine characteristics that naturally exist within them. This developmental task is often hampered by certain cultural influences and teachings, such as "Little boys don't cry" and "Little girls can't be angry." The gender-dominated professions of nursing and medicine, with their styles of relating and communicating frequently based on the feminine and masculine extremes described in Figure 7.1, make the capacity for achieving balance challenging for both nurses and physicians.

Balance is a characteristic of the 21st-century nurse, whether male or female. As Michael Williams concludes: "Nevertheless, I am convinced that bringing male and female perspectives equally to the point of care will enrich our profession and benefit our patients and families."

Potential Masculine Characteristics	Balanced Masculine and Feminine	Potential Feminine Characteristics
Anger	Emotional stability	Depression
Arrogance	Equality	Inferiority
Avoids showing vulnerability	Flexible	Avoids showing strength
Blaming	Learns from mistakes	Excusing
Ordering	Listening	Pleading
Denies feelings	In touch with feelings	Hysterical
Domineering	Creative	Victimized
Know-it-all	Curious	Knows nothing

Figure 7.1 The Masculine-Feminine Continuum

MEN + WOMEN AS NURSES = BALANCE

The fact that so few men are nurses has contributed to an interpersonal environment within the profession in which a nonassertive "feminine" extreme often represents its collective behavior, as documented in the professional literature. While there are outstanding exceptions to this among individuals and nursing groups, there is yet to be heard the proactive and unified voices of clarity and authority, which nurses are quite capable of expressing but are more typical of other professions, most notably medicine.

The men most dominant in the female nurse's professional life are usually not other nurses but rather physicians and administrators, who occupy positions of authority and power. While women also occupy these positions, they are fewer in number. It is an unfortunate reality that rather than working collaboratively, the nursing and medical professions frequently work hierarchically. The physician is in the dominant role, frequently expressing the behaviors characteristic of the masculine extremes noted in Figure 7.1, while the nurse typically is implicitly expected to behave in ways more closely aligned with characteristics representative of the feminine extreme. This has been and continues to be a major source of conflict for nurses, contributing to stressful work environments. It would be hard to find a nurse who hasn't had a firsthand experience and/or been witness to a physician's disruptive behavior, often aimed at a nurse and rarely dealt with effectively, if at all, by administrators.

Alan H. Rosenstein, MD, MBA, the physician-author of an important study titled "Nurse-Physician Relationships: Impact on Nurse Satisfaction and Retention" published in the June 2002 issue of *American Journal of Nursing*, at that time the official publication of the American Nurses Association (*nursingcenter.com*), corroborates this. The study surveyed nurses about their experiences with and perceptions of the physicians they worked with. It concluded that disruptive physician behavior and the institutional response to it do indeed affect nurses' morale.

Rosenstein verifies that "some of the issues of concern to nurses are deeply entrenched in the male-dominated physician and administrative cultures of hospitals, in which nursing is viewed as a subservient role and disruptive physician behavior is tolerated."[24] In an editorial that discusses the study, Diana Mason, PhD, RN, FAAN, the editor-in-chief of the *American Journal of Nursing*, called the nurse-physician relationships a "tired old dance, mired in gender inequity and historic precedent." She called the survey's physician-author "courageous" for discussing it and called on nurses to take responsibility for their role in perpetuating it by "changing their own steps."[25] One way, among many, that the power structure in healthcare might be influenced and equalized is by an increase in the number of men in nursing and women in medicine.

THE WOUND DRESSER

Walt Whitman's perceptions of the sufferings of the men he cared for as a nurse, as well as his efforts on their behalf, are described in his moving poem "The Wound Dresser." Read these sections from the poem and allow them to shatter what Michael Williams called "the most devaluing [myth] of all, the perception that a man cannot be caring and compassionate enough to be a nurse."

The Wound Dresser

Bearing the bandages, water and sponge,
Straight and swift to my wounded I go,
Where they lie on the ground after the battle brought in,
Where their priceless blood reddens the grass, the ground,
Or, to the rows of the hospital tent, or under the roof's hospital,
To the long rows of cots up and down each side I return,
To each and all one after another I draw near, not one do I miss,
An attendant follows holding a tray, he carries a refuse pail,

Soon to be filled with clotted rags and blood, emptied, and fill'd again.

I onward go, I stop,
With hinged knees and steady hand to dress wounds,
I am firm with each, the pangs are sharp yet avoidable,
One turns to me his appealing eyes—poor boy! I never knew you,
Yet I think I could not refuse this moment to die for you, if that would save you.

On, on I go (open doors of time! Open hospital doors!)
The crush'd head I dress, (poor crazed hand tear not the bandage away),
The neck of the cavalry-man with the bullet through and through I examine,
Hard the breathing rattles, quite glazed already the eye, yet life struggles hard,
(Come sweet death! Be persuaded O beautiful death! In mercy come quickly!)

From the stump of the arm, the amputated hand,
I undo the clotted lint, remove the slough,
Wash off the matter and blood,
Back on his pillow the soldier bends with
Curv'd neck and side falling head,
His eyes are closed, his face is pale, he
Dares not look on the bloody stump,
And has not yet look'd on it.

—Walt Whitman[26]

PART TWO

Converting Your Nursing Career into *You, Inc.*

CHAPTER 8

Becoming the Nurse CEO of *You, Inc.*

In 1996, at the height of the organizational restructuring and downsizing that helped shape the landscape of today's healthcare industry, William Bridges, author *of Job Shift: How to Prosper in a Workplace Without Jobs,* advocated a whole new way of looking at work and employment. He described a paradigm shift, a way to reframe how to think about work, which continues to be essential advice. He advised workers everywhere to manage their careers by converting themselves into a business and "to see yourself as a self-contained economic entity, not as a component part looking for a whole within which you can function."[1] This means shifting your thinking from having only a job (which by nature is owned by your employer) to owning your very transportable work skills and competencies. To see yourself as a self-contained economic entity means that your mental attitude is one of self-employment, whether you work for others or for yourself. This shift in thinking fosters the sense of empowerment and autonomy employers are seeking and is needed for ease of employability in rapidly changing workplaces. The following ways of thinking about your work expand on Bridge's advice:

- Be "vendor minded." In nursing practice, this would translate into being "consumer oriented," recognizing that everyone—the patient, your coworkers, your employer, and, of course, yourself—are consumers. This also captures the essence of nursing: the relationship with your patient.
- See yourself surrounded by a marketplace, with limitless options, whether or not you are on the payroll of an organization.
- Join, rather than blindly work for, your organization and customers (employers). This means selecting your employer carefully to ensure the best fit for your skills and competencies.

- Think like an entrepreneur—or, in the case of the employed nurse, an "intrapreneur"—by identifying or creating new work opportunities.
- Be independent as well as interdependent, relying on yourself as well as collaborating with others.
- Find new and creative ways to contribute your skills and competencies in current and emerging healthcare marketplaces.
- Commit to continuous learning.
- Create meaningful work, believing in the contribution you have to make.

Bridges was not a lone voice in this seemingly unconventional world of reframing how to think about jobs and work. Also in 1996, *U.S. News and World Report,* a mainstream publication, devoted 32 pages to an article entitled "You, Inc." The article described how all U.S. industries, including healthcare

> have leapt headlong into the information age, and how careers will never again be the same.... At no time in modern history have so many workers been so totally reliant on their own wits and resources to thrive.... The upshot: "You, Inc." may be the fastest growing employment segment in the economy, as people learn to invest in themselves as if they were a corporation.[2]

Invest in yourself as if you were a corporation! What a concept! What an empowering phrase! What would *your* work, *your* life, look like if you were to take this phrase and apply it seriously to your nursing career—if you considered yourself as the chief executive officer (CEO) of *You, Inc.?* And likewise, how would not investing in all aspects of your nursing "business" with the seriousness of a CEO affect your employability, your career mobility, and your professional satisfaction?

The nurse who is qualified to be the CEO of *You, Inc.* has the professional and personal characteristics that appear on the following page.

NURSE CEO OF *YOU, INC.*

PROFESSIONAL AND PERSONAL CHARACTERISTICS

Professional Experience and Characteristics

- Possesses targeted, progressive, cumulative work experience as a generalist and/or as a specialist.
- Can articulate examples of work experiences that have added value to the workplace.
- Is aware of, able to support, and can contribute to patient-focused care in a consumer-oriented business environment.
- Develops transferable skills.
- Is cross-trained.
- Seeks continuing education.
- Is comfortable with technology, including computers and the Internet.
- Possess or expects to obtain the Bachelor of Science in Nursing.
- Pursues advanced educational preparation commensurate with career goals.
- Receives ANCC board certification as a generalist or specialist or another professional certification.
- Seeks professional membership.

Personal Characteristics

- Is flexible, adaptive, assertive, confident, empowered.
- Is both self-directed and team oriented.
- Strives to be an innovative problem solver.
- Does not accept the status quo.
- Is willing to take risks.
- Learns from mistakes.
- Resolves conflicts.
- Thinks critically.
- Is a master networker, online and in person.

The primary mission of *You, Inc.* evolves from periodic reflection and exploration of the following questions:

- Are the skills and competencies you have to offer (your nursing "business") current with respect to the needs of healthcare employers?
- What makes you stand out from others seeking the same opportunity?
- What contributions are you making to the mission of your current employer? Or what are you willing to offer a potential employer?
- In what ways does your current employer contribute to the mission of *You, Inc.*—to the skills and competencies it needs? Is it supporting your professional and personal growth?
- In what ways have you or will you improve the quality of service that the organization provides, over and above the minimum requirement of showing up for work and performing the tasks required in the job description?

These questions are important, because healthcare operates in a managed care environment where organizational viability is driven by the bottom line. If a particular activity (a nursing role, for example) cannot be translated into direct or indirect profit, it cannot continue unchanged if the organization is to survive. Harsh as this may sound, this does not have to be mutually exclusive with caring for and about patients. More importantly, it is seen by your employer as *the way* to care, as a road map for providing high-quality patient care, as long as it is tempered with best practices and sound ethical and moral standards. Since this is a reality in today's healthcare marketplace, it needs to be a reality for *You, Inc.* as well.

To manage and administer *You, Inc.* most effectively, you need to know the ways in which your business—your product/service, if you will—is different from that of others. You also need to be proactive enough to express these personal and professional attributes in performance appraisals, on your resume, during interviews, and so on. You should aim to get as close as you can to having the professional experiences and personal characteristics described below. You should have a plan for developing those attributes you don't yet have, seeing *You, Inc.* as a work in progress, and evolving within the same kind of continuous quality improvement as the healthcare organizations for which you are working.

The Nurse CEO of *You, Inc.*

Organization or Corporation	***You, Inc.***
Has a mission statement, a clearly stated purpose.	Has a mission statement aligned with values and a vision.
Has an operating license.	Has an RN license and perhaps others.
Is insured against malpractice.	Carries malpractice insurance and accidental injury claims and other insurance as indicated.
Operates based on written standards of practice.	Utilizes ANA Standards in the practice of nursing.
Abides by ethical standards.	Abides by the ANA Code of Ethics.
Utilizes policies and procedures for the delivery of its services and the fulfillment of its mission.	Develops policies and procedures that determine where, when, and for how long *You, Inc.* will provide its services in a particular segment of the healthcare marketplace.
Engages in continuous quality improvement programs.	Engages in continuous training and education to improve the quality and marketability of skills and services.
Seeks and applies for recognition by associations and accrediting agencies for outstanding achievement and excellence in service, such as Magnet Hospital Status awarded by ANCC.	Seeks out recognition for professional achievement through ANCC board certification or through other professional associations. Uses Magnet Hospital Status as one criterion for choosing employment.
Builds alliances, coalitions, networks, and partnerships with other organizations.	Considers itself a partner to healthcare organizations. The organization has patients that need healthcare services; *You, Inc.* provides those services and builds professional and personal networks.
Competes effectively with other organizations that provide the same service by means of effective marketing and public relations.	Adapts business strategies to position *You, Inc.* to compete effectively, including product development, market research, advertising (resume), sales (interviewing), networking strategies, and the development of a marketing plan.

As you compare the two lists on page 131, you may recognize that most of the expectations and functions necessary for *You, Inc.* aren't too different from what has always been expected of nurses who want to excel, except perhaps for the last item about utilizing business strategies as a career management tool.

To make this shift, think of yourself as the CEO of *You, Inc.* with your own headquarters of operation in an office in your home or just in your mind's eye. From this place, you can plan, implement, and track the activities of *You, Inc.*, as well as oversee, coordinate, and manage the departments of *You, Inc.* listed in figure 8.1.

Department	Responsibilities and Functions
Product Development	Develops and communicates what *You, Inc* has to offer: its mission statement (skills, competencies, experience, transferable skills), vision, and values.
Market Research	Conducts ongoing research to determine where along the continuum of care *You, Inc.*'s nursing skills and competencies are most needed; determines how best to take advantage of newly emerging healthcare opportunities.
Advertising	Creates and revises *You, Inc.*'s resume and maintains a professional portfolio.
Sales	Develops and hones techniques for interviewing effectively in order to "sell" *You, Inc.*'s nursing skills and competencies.
Networking	Creates and maintains professional and personal alliances and relationships through fluid use of online and in person experiences.
Marketing Plan	Performs ongoing assessments of needs and develops strategic career plans with defined goals, stated tasks, and specific timelines.

Figure 8.1

THE CONTINUUM OF WORK

To develop the kind of self-employed attitude that has been described requires a mental shift, a way to reframe how you think about your work even though you are officially an employee. You can do this in the following ways:

- Reconceptualize the manner in which you describe your work and where it falls on the "Continuum of Work." (See figure 8.2.)
- Recognize that the employer owns the job you do, while you own your very portable work and ever-expanding transferable skills.
- Aim for empowered mutuality and interdependence in your work relationships, instead of allowing yourself to be passively dependent or overreliant on the direction of others.

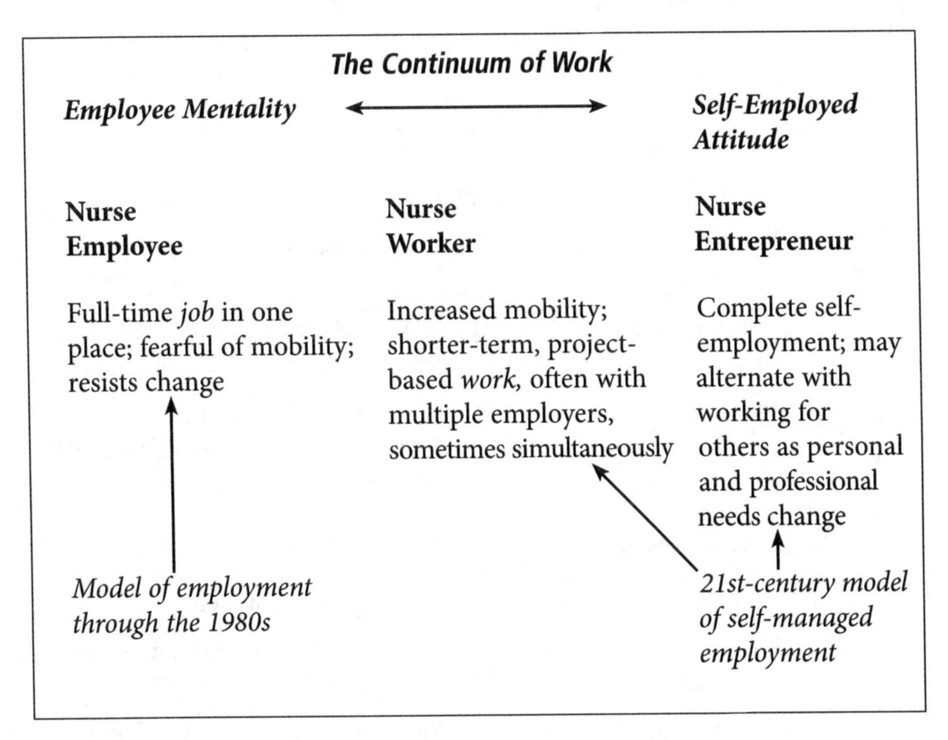

Figure 8.2

EMPOWERMENT AND THE NEW EMPLOYMENT CONTRACT

To be empowered is to act on your own behalf. Empowerment is the essence of the self-employed attitude; it is what fuels the actions of the nurse CEO of *You, Inc.* To be empowered is the refusal to be trapped without options—no matter what. Empowerment means staying loyal to yourself, your needs and values, your professional and personal mission and vision, while simultaneously committing yourself to the goals of the organization while you are employed there. It's a tall order but essential nonetheless.

To be empowered is to remember that your work is portable: it belongs to you, while the job you are occupying belongs to your employer and will remain there when you leave with your accumulated work experience in tow. Twenty-first century employers are expecting a more mobile and autonomous workforce, representing a shift in the employer-employee relationship that has existed since the Industrial Revolution. Influenced by a new understanding that today's complex workplace requires mutuality and collaboration rather than the hierarchical decision making of the past, a new employment contract is emerging, with employers expecting a much more self-directed and empowered employee. This shift in thinking, which has important implications for career planning, is well described by David Noer in *Healing the Wounds.*[3] Below is a summary of his thoughts.

- **Old employment contract:**
  - Tenure and long-term relationships
  - Linear promotion as reward for performance within fixed job descriptions
  - Loyalty to and lifetime employment at the organization, which provides long-term career paths and discourages external hiring
  - A workforce that was potentially older, nondiverse, plateaued, demotivated, codependent, and mediocre with limited potential for empowerment
- **New employment contract:**
  - Situational employment with flexible, portable benefit plans
  - Blurred distinction between full-time, part-time, and temporary employees
  - Rewards for performance based on tenure-free acknowledgment of contribution achieved through self-directed work teams and nonhierarchical performance systems
  - More autonomous employees
  - Loyalty meaning responsibility and good work within nontraditional career paths
  - A mobile workforce that is flexible, motivated, task invested, empowered, and responsible

Understanding this new employment relationship will allow you greater flexibility in managing your career, especially in the context of the cost-containment influences of managed care. Healthcare systems will continue to reorganize themselves and restructure roles to reduce costs. An example that could easily affect you is the merger of two medical centers. Suppose you were a nurse on an inpatient pediatric unit in a large metropolitan medical center that has just merged with another, which also has a full-service pediatric center. The initial response as the CEO of *You, Inc.* should be to conduct marketplace research to determine which pediatric services are now being duplicated and which will possibly be reorganized. This analysis will begin to give you the information you need to determine how best to position yourself in this new environment, or if you even want to, knowing that roles and responsibilities are likely to change.

The Empowerment Continuum

As you might imagine, the most empowered behaviors correlate with a self-employed attitude. Think about empowerment as an active process in which you learn to engage in skillful behaviors that contribute to an assertive and proactive expression of yourself. Ensuring that you have role models that embody empowerment allows you to see this in action. Give yourself permission to imitate or "borrow" their behavior to make it your own over time.

Another way to conceptualize empowerment is on a continuum, with the least empowered behaviors occurring on one end and the most empowered behaviors occurring on the other. This empowerment continuum (see figure 8.3) can be a useful professional growth tool, serving as a guide to your professional development and as a way to benchmark, or measure, your success. During this nursing shortage cycle, when nurses are being asked to do so much more with fewer and fewer resources, the capacity to say no to unreasonable requests and to advocate for your own well-being has never been more important. This is the essence of the empowered nurse who is not only acting on her or his own behalf but ensuring safe patient care as well. For more about empowerment, including the process of cultivating it, see chapter 15.

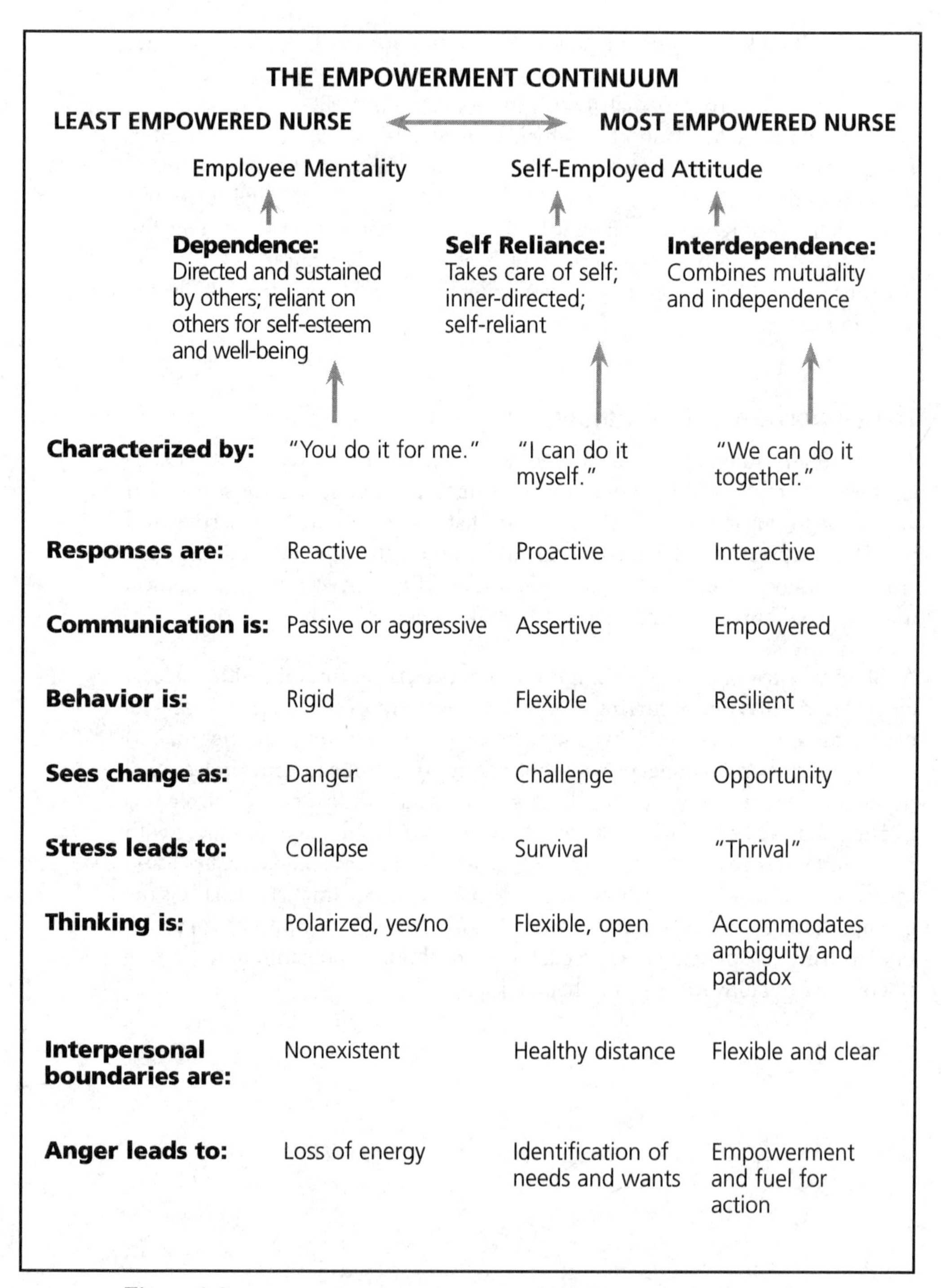
THE EMPOWERMENT CONTINUUM
LEAST EMPOWERED NURSE
MOST EMPOWERED NURSE
Employee Mentality
Self-Employed Attitude
Dependence: Directed and sustained by others; reliant on others for self-esteem and well-being
Self Reliance: Takes care of self; inner-directed; self-reliant
Interdependence: Combines mutuality and independence
Characterized by:
"You do it for me."
"I can do it myself."
"We can do it together."
Responses are:
Reactive
Proactive
Interactive
Communication is:
Passive or aggressive
Assertive
Empowered
Behavior is:
Rigid
Flexible
Resilient
Sees change as:
Danger
Challenge
Opportunity
Stress leads to:
Collapse
Survival
"Thrival"
Thinking is:
Polarized, yes/no
Flexible, open
Accommodates ambiguity and paradox
Interpersonal boundaries are:
Nonexistent
Healthy distance
Flexible and clear
Anger leads to:
Loss of energy
Identification of needs and wants
Empowerment and fuel for action

Figure 8.3

PROFILE OF A NURSE CEO OF *YOU, INC.*

Debbie, a single parent of a two-year-old daughter, works as a fee-for-service (per diem) home care nurse in two home care agencies simultaneously. She pays for her own and her daughter's health and disability insurance and has recently established a private retirement fund managed by a financial advisor at her local bank.

She is an ANCC-certified medical-surgical nurse practicing at the generalist level and will soon complete an adult nurse practitioner program paid for by scholarships, savings targeted for starting school, and one low-interest student loan. Her role at the home care agencies is aligned with her work values of autonomy and independence, and it supports *You, Inc.*'s mission of "influencing and supporting the physical and emotional health of older adults." Her long-term vision is to create more in-home mental health services, especially for the isolated homebound patients who make up the majority of her practice and for whom very little mobile support is available. She is a member of the Telenursing Committee, which is about to implement remote monitoring of patients' blood pressure and glucose levels using a cell phone–based system.

Debbie arranges her work schedule and maintains an income so as to support her school goals and parenting responsibilities by reducing the number of hours she is available to agencies when school is in session and increasing them during semester breaks. She is careful about the kind of assignments she accepts when she is in school, reducing her caseload when necessary.

Debbie self-manages the components of work life traditionally managed by employers, including health and disability insurance, retirement savings, tuition reimbursement, time scheduling, and patient assignments. She carries her own malpractice insurance. She misses the natural relationship building that goes on in workplaces where people are in the same building all day, but she substitutes school-based involvement when classes are in session and tries to attend professional meetings during semester breaks. She also utilizes online social networking sites to establish and maintain personal and professional contacts.

Debbie embodies the work skills as well as the self-directed, empowered, and collaborative attitude employers are looking for today. She is the kind of employee to whom they expect to extend an employment contract suited to this century's workplace realities.

CHAPTER 9

The Product Development Department of *You, Inc.*

Your nursing skills and competencies, your experience, and your transferable skills all comprise the "product" you have to offer/sell to potential employers, who then utilize this "product" to provide services that benefit their customers/ patients. Even though the nurse is providing a service, not a product per se, we will use the term *product* for ease in discussing the business application of this work activity. Considering your work as a nurse in this manner is not mutually exclusive from your professional image, and it does not interfere with the relationships you establish with your patients. Rather, this way of thinking provides you with a model within which to shape and guide your career.

YOUR PRODUCT

For your product to be most attractive to the healthcare employers of your choice and for your own satisfaction, two areas of product development require your focus: professional development and personal development. Chapter 15 ("The Resilient You") will provide you with an opportunity to explore your personal development. This chapter will give you ideas on how to strengthen your professional development.

The state of rapid change and permanent transition that characterized the downsizing era of the 1990s is the new status quo. Expect your professional and personal lives to be fluid, to change unexpectedly, and to require fast adaptation. Recognizing this will allow you to position *You, Inc.* to take best advantage of opportunities as the healthcare marketplace continues to shift.

When change affects your job responsibilities, you have at least two options. The first is to realign your product by updating your skills to those now required. The second is to offer your original product where it is still needed. For example, suppose you are an operating room (OR) nurse in a hospital that merged with another from across town and will offer surgical services only at that location. This newly formed medical center now finds itself with far too many OR nurses and has offered you a transfer to its Cardiac Intervention Center, which will be expanding to accommodate more patients. You could choose to remain an OR nurse and offer your product to another employer, or you could choose to use this as an opportunity to add cardiac skills to your product.

In this era, it is possible that a marketplace shift significant enough to affect your work could occur about every six months. Changes could come from movement in the healthcare system itself or a related shift in society, which in turn influences the healthcare industry. To keep current and stay aligned with changes that will occur in your work or personal life, you need to conduct periodic, perhaps biannual, assessments of the current state and marketability of your product. Look at the three questions below. Reflecting on the answers to these queries (and recognizing that the answers will change over time) will ensure optimal mobility and career satisfaction.

1. Who are you as a nurse? How are you the same as or different from other nurses?
2. What do you have to offer? Describe your product.
3. Who needs your product? Target your market; identify your employer.

In this chapter, we will explore the answers to the first two questions. The third question will be discussed in chapter 10.

WHO ARE YOU?

You are unique; you are complex. Your needs and preferences may be similar to those of others, but you blend those needs differently than anyone else in the world. Who you are as a nurse is certainly more than the job you do. Which of the following descriptions most closely resembles how you think about your nursing practice?

- **Nursing is my job:** It belongs to someone else (the employer). It is given to me for a period of time, the length of which is not necessarily determined by me and can be modified at the will of my employer, not always with my input or permission.
- **Nursing is my work:** It is a use of my learned skills, competencies, and experience, often by mutual agreement with an employer. It

> is based on my life purpose, guided by my vision, grounded in my values, and frequently expressed in a series of temporary work experiences called jobs.

The nurse CEO of *You, Inc.* knows the difference between work and job as well as how they relate to each other. Your job represents your current professional focus within an ever-evolving career of highly portable work experiences. Your work reflects your mission (your purpose in life), which is rooted in your values and your vision for how all this fits together.

Throughout your nursing career, as you periodically reflect on and refine the answers to who you are and what you have to offer, you will find yourself solidifying what is permanently yours—namely, your work. Owning your work in this manner enhances career satisfaction, deters burnout, and strengthens your ability to withstand the winds of change, whether in the healthcare industry or elsewhere in your life.

Think about your nursing career as symbolized by a strong, firmly rooted oak tree. Imagine that its branches represent your evolving vision growing, expanding, and reaching upward. The leaves on the tree represent your current skills and competencies, which are renewed annually when old "leaves" fall away and new replacements follow. The strong trunk of the tree holds your mission—your purpose—acting as a kind of rudder to steady and guide your career, even when the winds of change blow the branches about. Your values are represented by the deep roots of the tree held firmly by the soil in which the tree is planted. The soil is the marketplace, which turns over periodically, losing or gaining nutrients. Water, symbolizing ongoing training, education, and self-care, nourishes the tree and supports its growth. Fertilizer and nutrients for the tree come in the form of mentors, preceptors, and others who provide support, guidance, and advice. In summary, each aspect of the tree represents an area requiring your focus to ensure alignment of your product with current marketplace needs. This includes your vision, mission, values, skills, competencies, and self-care.

YOUR MISSION

An ad for a major New York medical center read as follows: "Providing compassionate quality healthcare isn't our job … it's our mission." Likewise, while *You, Inc.* may occupy a job slot for a particular employer for a certain length of time, it does so to enact its mission, which hopefully is aligned with that of the employer.

Developing Your Mission

A mission is the evolving expression of what you believe your life purpose to be. It is based on innate as well as learned abilities. It includes preferences for life activities (including those outside of work) that are rooted in your value system and aligned with your vision. In her book *The Path,* Laurie Beth Jones describes a mission statement as

> a written-down reason for being; key to finding your path in life and to identifying the mission you choose to follow; having a clearly articulated mission statement gives one a template of purpose that can be used to initiate, evaluate, and refine all of one's activities.[1]

What is your "written-down reason for being," your "template of purpose"? Determining this is essential to forming a strong foundation upon which to build *You, Inc.* This becomes a way to keep yourself grounded even as you move forward—or a way to decide not to move in a particular direction with which your mission is not aligned.

Jones says that finding your mission and then fulfilling it is "perhaps the most vital activity in which a person can engage." Steven Covey, author of *The 7 Habits of Highly Effective People* and *First Things First,* echoes this. Covey describes a mission statement as follows:

> A philosophy or creed which focuses on what you want to be (character) and do (contributions and achievements), and on the values (principles) upon which being and doing is based; it is a written standard, a personal constitution, and like the United States Constitution, based on self-evident truths of the Declaration of Independence; it is fundamentally changeless, defended and supported, pledged allegiance to, and enables people to ride through such major traumas as war; it empowers individuals with tireless strength in the midst of change.[2]

So many phrases in Covey's description of a mission statement have relevance to your nursing career and to *You, Inc.* For example, pledging allegiance to yourself rather than your employer keeps you free to stay or go, depending on which way the winds of change are blowing and, most importantly, whether the change is still aligned with your mission.

In 1995, during the height of the downsizing crisis, Leah Curtin, editor of *Nursing Management*, captured the meaning of this for nurses of that time. Her thoughts are still quite relevant today. She said:

> Nurses must learn to redirect their loyalty from their employer to their work, committing themselves to self-development and skills enlargement. As they invest in themselves, they become more valuable.

Where is your loyalty? To whom are you pledging allegiance? And how is it affecting your ability to declare yourself independent? While your employer certainly warrants your commitment to its mission for the length of time you choose to stay, your loyalty and allegiance belong to *You, Inc.* What "self-evident truths" are in your personal "constitution"? What will you battle over, stand up for, defend, and support—no matter what? For example, in what ways might *You, Inc.* stand up for, defend, and support safe staffing ratios, adequate time for meal breaks, and the elimination of mandatory overtime?

Thinking about Your Mission Statement

A mission statement is not something you write overnight or in one sitting. Rather, it evolves over time. According to Covey, it takes "deep introspection, careful analysis, and thoughtful expression" as you reflect on where you've been and how it has affected you, where you want to go, and what you want your life to be about. Because it is a solid expression of your values and vision, it should not be written in isolation from them. Jones describes the elements of a mission statement as these:

- No longer than a single sentence
- Easily understood by a 12-year-old
- Able to be recited automatically, by memory
- Perfectly suited to you

In both the Covey and Jones books, you will find excellent descriptions and exercises to use in developing your mission statement (see Endnotes at the back of this book). Use the following exercise, adapted from *The Path,* to get started.

There are three steps to creating your mission statement:

Step 1: What you do, expressed in three action verbs

Step 2: What you stand for; the principles, causes you would defend to the death; your core value or values

Step 3: Who you want to help; who you really want to serve, be around, inspire, learn from, impact, and make a difference for

Step 1

Select three words from the list of action verbs below that most excite you, shed light on who you are, and describe what you most like to spend your time doing. (This is a partial list based on a more complete one in *The Path.*)

facilitate	foster	alleviate
prepare	realize	communicate
improve	involve	motivate
educate	support	empower
sustain	enhance	organize

Write the three words representing what you do here:

________ ________ ________

Step 2

Write a word or key phrase that describes your core value or values, the principle or principles you would defend to the death, such as *joy* or *service* or *justice* or *independence*. (For additional value words, consult the list in the self-assessment exercise that begins on page 148.)

Write what you stand for here: ____

Step 3

Describe those whom you want to help—the more specific, the better. Consider the kind of healthcare client, the patient population or nursing specialty, the age group, and so on.

Write whom you help here: ____

Creating Your Mission Statement

Combine the words from Steps 1, 2, and 3 to form your mission statement. Fill in the blanks below:

My mission (what I do):

____________________, ____________________, and ____________________

(your three action verbs from Step 1)

My values or principles (what I stand for):

____

(your core values or principles from Step 2)

To or for, among or with (those whom you help):

____

(the group or cause from Step 3)

Sample Mission Statement: John

John, a direct care nurse in a family health clinic, wrote the following mission statement, which helped him determine where to look for his next work experience upon learning that the clinic had lost its grant funding and would have to close.

My mission (what I do):

nurture, educate, and facilitate

My values or principles (what I stand for):

health and well-being

To or for, among or with (those whom you help):

traditional and nontraditional families, including single fathers

Having this as his mission statement helped John recognize that the employer could take away only his job—not his work, not his career, and certainly not his mission. It helped him to focus on what he wanted his next career experience to be and what employer might be most interested in the work he had to offer. Within two months, he was working as a visiting nurse, making home visits to new moms and dads, many of whom were young and engaging in high-risk behaviors.

Here are some additional examples of mission statements representative of the work nurses do:

- Facilitate, teach, and encourage the mental and emotional health of inner-city school children.
- Inspire, recognize, and promote healing in grieving adults.
- Communicate, demonstrate, and encourage computer literacy among healthcare professionals.
- Model, nurture, and facilitate empowerment in single mothers.

- Inspire, improve, and sustain self-care and independence in "the oldest old" (people over 85).
- Develop, prepare, and circulate diabetic teaching materials for newly diagnosed children.

YOUR VALUES AND NEEDS

Values are the beliefs that ground your decisions and activities in the work world and in your personal life. They are the expression of deeply held beliefs about how you like things to be and what you prefer to experience. Values are often based on and influenced by psychological needs. Examples of values include to be with people, to be independent, to be useful, to experience stability, to have influence, to serve others, and so on. (See in the self-assessment exercise that begins on page 148 for an expanded list of values.)

Values shape your interests and influence which skills you decide to learn as well as the accomplishments you achieve. Because your values and needs form the basis of the personal interests you pursue and the career paths you select, knowing about them is essential to the question, *Who are you?*

Take Orinthia, for example, who currently works in the newborn nursery of a community hospital. She has worked in this hospital for four years, and this is her third assignment in the obstetrical department, where nurses rotate for six-month periods to each clinical area, including the ambulatory care clinics. Orinthia is experiencing the same kind of boredom and restlessness that she remembers having twice before, once when she worked on the postpartum unit and, before that, when she worked in the prenatal clinic. The one time during this current rotation that she remembered feeling genuinely interested in her work was when it was decided that infants experiencing mild respiratory distress would no longer be transferred out to the neonatal intensive care unit (NICU) of a major medical center for treatment. Instead, the nurses in the newborn nursery would be taught the skills needed to care for these infants. She learned the assessment and technical skills quickly and, in fact, became a resource to two of her nurse colleagues, Barbara and Joan, who initially found these critical care tasks overwhelming. When these nurses investigated what values and needs might be represented by their preferences for work assignments, it became clear that there were some striking differences among them. Orinthia identified the following needs and values as important to her:

Challenge: Work that is mentally stimulating

Detail work: Performance of tasks requiring accurate focus and attention

Fast pace: Meet demanding expectations within time deadlines

Excitement: Work characterized by frequent novelty and drama

Variety: Frequent change in job responsibilities

Barbara and Joan, the nurses who felt overwhelmed by this new assignment, identified the following values and needs:

Predictability: Satisfaction with routine, repetitious tasks

Expertise: Being good at something

Mastery: Acquired proficiency and expertise in tasks

Connection: Giving and receiving care, support, and warmth

While all three nurses loved working with mothers and babies, Orinthia preferred caring for the sicker infants, while her peers did not. In addition, Orinthia realized that she had experienced practically none of the work preferences representative of her values and needs during her past rotations to the postpartum unit or the prenatal clinic; her work preferences were only present in this current rotation when she was assigned to care for these sick infants. During those times, she felt challenged by the potential unpredictability of the sick infant's health status and the fast-paced work requiring attention to detail that was missing for her in the routine care of well babies, exactly what her peers enjoyed.

After these nurses identified their needs and values in relation to the kind of work they preferred, they were able to request work assignments that resulted in more professional satisfaction and experienced less boredom and stress. Orinthia was assigned to care for the infants with respiratory distress whenever possible, while the other nurses performed the tasks more routinely associated with well baby care, including the teaching and emotional support of new parents.

Eventually, Orinthia went to work in the obstetrical department of a hospital that didn't require rotation through all the ob-gyn subspecialties and was permanently assigned to the NICU, where the fast pace suited her perfectly and was aligned with her mission to "support, facilitate, or strengthen connection in the mother-baby bond of critically ill newborns."

Complete the exercise on the following page to begin exploring and clarifying your needs and values as they relate to your work preferences, your mission, your vision, and the larger question of *Who are you?* (Adapted from James C. Cabrera and Charles F. Albrecht Jr., *The Lifetime Career Manager: New Strategies for a New Era* [Cincinnati, OH: Adams Media Corporation, 1997].)[3]

SELF-ASSESSMENT EXERCISE: YOUR NEEDS AND VALUES

Rank the following needs and values and their descriptions according to the following scale:

1 = Always necessary. Impossible or very hard to work or live without.

2 = Often necessary. Could work or live without it, if necessary, or temporarily, but wouldn't want to; would miss it a lot.

3 = Sometimes necessary. Would prefer to have it, but could manage fairly well if it wasn't there.

4 = Rarely or never necessary. Could easily work or live without it; don't think about it much.

Score	Value	Description
_____	Achievement	Attain and maintain a sense of accomplishment mastery.
_____	Aesthetics	Work in a setting that values the beauty of things and ideas.
_____	Affection	Express and receive warmth and caring.
_____	Authenticity	Be genuinely yourself.
_____	Balance	Achieve satisfactory proportion between work and personal life.
_____	Career advancement	Experience opportunities for vertical mobility (promotion), as well as horizontal mobility (transfer), within the workplace.
_____	Challenge	Experience work as mentally stimulating.
_____	Competition	Achieve mastery by competing with others or by challenging yourself.
_____	Creativity	Express imagination and ingenuity in work.
_____	Detail work	Perform tasks requiring accurate focus and detail.
_____	Efficient organization	Work in an organization that runs effectively with minimal bureaucracy.

(Go on to next page.)

SELF-ASSESSMENT EXERCISE (CONT.)

_____	Excitement	Experience adventure, frequent novelty, and drama.
_____	Expertise	Feeling skilled, being good at something.
_____	Emotional resilience	Ability to mediate and process personal feelings and bounce back from interpersonal difficulties.
_____	Fast pace	Meet demanding expectations within time deadlines.
_____	Family	Experience contented personal relationships or living situation.
_____	Friendship	Develop social and personal relationships with peers and colleagues.
_____	Health	Pursue physical, mental, and emotional well-being.
_____	Helping others	Contribute to or assist others in need.
_____	Independence	Control the type of work you do, including schedule.
_____	Integrity	Work ethically and honestly.
_____	Knowledge	Learn and use specific information.
_____	Leadership	Influence, authorize, or direct others to achieve results.
_____	Location	Live in a convenient geographical location in a suitable community.
_____	Management	Achieve work goals as a result of the efforts of others.
_____	Money	Reap significant financial rewards.
_____	Meaningful work	Perform work that has purpose, relevance.

(Go on to next page.)

SELF-ASSESSMENT EXERCISE (CONT.)

_____	Personal growth	Develop and grow into your potential.
_____	Pleasure	Experience enjoyment, fun, satisfaction.
_____	Physical health	Express vitality and well-being.
_____	Positive atmosphere	Work in a pleasing, supportive, harmonious setting.
_____	Power	Control the resources at work.
_____	Recognition	Receive credit and appreciation for work well done; be known or well known; be praised.
_____	Security	Work without fear of unemployment, have stable future.
_____	Service	Contribute to the well-being, welfare, or satisfaction of another.
_____	Spirituality	Express meaning of life or religious beliefs.
_____	Status	Attain a position of recognized importance.
_____	Variety and change	Perform tasks of great variety.
_____	Wisdom	Develop insight and understanding.
_____	Work with others	Belong to a satisfying work group or team.

Interpreting Your Score

In reviewing this self-assessment, notice how many 1s and 2s you have. The 1s and 2s relate to values and needs that should not be compromised—at least not for long—because compromising them can lead to personal and interpersonal conflict, stress, and eventually burnout. The 3s and 4s are places where you can allow more compromise as you attempt to align *You, Inc.* with the reality of any given situation.

You may be living out of balance, in disharmony, with who you are if your values and needs are blocked from expression. While it is unrealistic to expect the workplace to match all of your needs and values, a preponderance of them should be met for you to feel satisfied and productive. A value system that is very misaligned with the work you are doing is a prescription for stress. Should you find yourself in this situation, consider the following options.

Options for Addressing Unmet Values

Compensate for Your Unmet Values

Compensate for missing values by identifying other places for their expression. Perhaps you could take courses, enroll in seminars, join a support group, or engage in a personal inquiry through psychotherapy.

Negotiate for Your Values

Negotiate for the value or need that is not being fulfilled. For example, if you scored a 1 or 2 for the need for recognition and it is in short supply where you work, try asking for feedback more often or consider participating in a work activity that might provide some consistent appreciation for a job well done, perhaps committee work.

Realign Your Values

This does not mean giving up what keeps you rooted in the essence of who you are. Rather, to realign your values means to evaluate what your current job can realistically provide and see if you can modify your expectations accordingly. This might be possible if you know that your job is temporary or if you design your personal life so that it offers ample opportunities for the expression of the needs or values blocked at work.

For example, if you scored a 1 or 2 for "power" (controlling resources at work) and this is not possible within your current job responsibilities, try relating to what is there, not what you wish could be, and learn to let go of what you cannot control. This could be a growth experience for you as you learn to adjust and accommodate to the reality of your situation, rather than fighting to change the unchangeable. When you have not succeeded in changing something you don't like and you decide to stay in the situation anyway, you can find relief from the tension this creates by changing the way you think about it. Marcel Proust captured this idea well when he said:

> The real voyage of discovery consists not in seeking new landscapes but in having new eyes.

Where might you need to change how you think about or see something? Keep in mind that selecting this option requires paying very careful attention to the fine line between flexibility and total compromise of one's needs and values. Many nurses are faced with this dilemma because of the higher volume of sicker patients requiring care during shorter stays in these times of managed care and fiscal restraint. The phrase "do more with less" is an affront to the nursing profession's collective values regarding the provision of safe and ethical care, and individual nurses need to examine carefully what can be compromised and what cannot.

Another situation that might require some realignment of values is what you think or feel about healthcare employers utilizing business principles and philosophies to run their organizations. Is caring for others mutually exclusive from running a business? Is it possible to have a business/bottom-line mentality and still provide compassionate and empathic care? Coming to terms with this reality requires moving away from black-and-white, either-or thinking and finding a middle ground where the values of caring and business can coexist side by side. This kind of reframing and revisioning is necessary for complex issues like these, helping the nurse to discover the "new eyes" of which Proust wrote.

Honor and Stand Up for Your Values

Decide whether a career move, and perhaps a new career path, is necessary because your values are either too compromised or just cannot be met where you are. For example, if control of resources is essential to you and realigning your expectations is not possible, ask yourself why you're working in a place that can't meet these needs. If your answer has more to do with salary and employment benefits than your overall career goals, you might benefit from re-examining and prioritizing your needs and values with a mentor or coach who can provide objective feedback and guidance. If you believe that the latest changes in your workplace have made it impossible to provide safe, effective care, you would be better off working where your values and needs about patient care delivery could more easily be met.

Another way to stand up for what you believe in is to assist others in fighting for what you are not able to influence on your own. One example might be supporting the legislative efforts of your state nurses association as it addresses safe staffing guidelines and whistle-blower laws. Joining the American Nurses Association and participating directly through committee work or indirectly though membership dues is another way to honor and stand up for your nursing practice values.

DEVELOPING YOUR VISION

Robert Kennedy said, "Some men see things as they are and ask, 'Why?' I dream of the things that could be and ask, 'Why not?'" Kennedy had a vision of the future that he believed in. Do you? A vision of what you want for the immediate or even distant future is necessary for *You, Inc.* A vision is a place for your hopes and dreams to grow. It is a guidepost for your plans and goals. It is where your mission and your values will still make sense, even though they will be shaped and refined in the process of getting there.

Having a vision of the future provides a stabilizing anchor in the present that can steady you through turbulent times while serving as a beacon of hope and optimism toward which you navigate. A vision can become a powerful self-care and stress management strategy, because it prevents you from feeling trapped or victimized in a situation that may no longer be aligned with your mission or values. A vision gives you some realistic control over your destiny, especially if you use your present experience as a training ground to accumulate the skills and experiences that will transfer to what you envision yourself doing in the future.

For example, Clarissa values teaching and enjoys helping people feel more confident in their ability to learn complicated things. She has been working as a direct care nurse on a medical unit for four years and especially likes helping newly diagnosed diabetics feel less overwhelmed as they learn to manage their own care. Because of the nursing shortage, Clarissa has found herself with additional work assignments that allow her less time for teaching, even though this is still an expected part of her job.

In taking stock of her present situation, as well as what she envisions herself doing in the future, Clarissa imagines combining her nursing knowledge and the knack she has for teaching complicated concepts in understandable ways with her growing interest in technology, specifically computers and the Internet. She came across an article on the role of the informatics nurse and began imagining herself doing that kind of work. Exactly what she would be doing and where was vague, but the more she imagined it and allowed for the possibility of it, the more motivated she felt about exploring what it would take to make it happen.

When Clarissa heard that the hospital was offering advanced computer classes, she jumped at the chance to enroll. She also volunteered to work on a newly formed task force that was designing self-taught computer modules for patients. Her dissatisfaction with her current job was easier to tolerate, because she used every opportunity to add to the skills and competencies she believed were transferable to her future vision. She volunteered to assist in the development of standardized teaching plans to make the work of busy nurses easier. She found resources for and developed patient teaching kits with handouts that simplified concepts and saved time. As she was doing this, she pored over the want ads to learn what the qualifications were for informatics nurses, what kind of organizations employed them, and what educational preparation was required. She read everything she could get her hands on about this role, attended seminars about it, and eventually entered a graduate program that prepared nurses for it.

Clarissa used her vision to encourage her to move forward as she strengthened her mission and held tight to her values. In this way she made productive and creative use of an otherwise unacceptable employment situation.

Creating a vision relies primarily on the thinking style most closely associated with right-brain processes where thought occurs in mental impressions, fleeting images, and intuitive hunches. It is the twin partner of the logical processing and sequential reasoning associated with the capacities of the left brain. Using both of these processes results in a more complete picture of the future situation you are pondering. While considering your future with left-brain capacities leads to goals, tasks, and checklists, combining this with your right-brain abilities can encourage and even accelerate momentum toward your dreams and hopes.

Right-brain thought is rich with the information and the support needed to move into the future, but because rational reasoning is favored as the dominant thinking style of the scientifically based Western world, our right-brain abilities receive less training and validation. Creative right-brain activities are not always understood or encouraged. As a child, you may remember daydreaming (an essential function of creativity and vision building) and being told by a parent or teacher that you were not paying attention. Or perhaps you were told not to let your imagination "run away with you" as you wrote a story or spoke to an imaginary playmate. These normal, creative, and eminently useful right-brain thinking processes can be recaptured by devoting a little time and effort to relearning and remembering them and by suspending judgment and criticism of the process as well as the results.

Tips and Guidelines for Developing Your Vision

Write It Down

Write down your vision and recall it frequently. Say it aloud, to yourself at first, always using present tense vocabulary. Writing it down creates a kind of contract with yourself, and speaking about it in the present tense acts as a feedback loop to strengthen your resolve when the going gets tough. Share it with people who encourage and believe in you. Hearing yourself talk about it out loud reinforces the reality of it and helps move it from the possible to the probable, and eventually into the actual.

Take Your Vision Outside of Your Comfort Zone

Allow your vision to stretch you beyond your comfort zone without being unrealistic or overly ambitious. Marcia Perkins-Reed writes about vision in her book *Thriving in Transition*. She says the following:

> It [vision] should challenge us to reach further than we have before. If we do this at each of our transitional junctures, we will be constantly growing into greater possibilities. So if we think we can easily earn $45,000 in our next position, a minimum salary of $47,500 or $50,000 should appear in our vision statement. While we don't want to push ourselves relentlessly, ever striving towards elusive new goals that we don't believe will bring us success, we do want to expand our vision into the highest and best situation we can imagine, knowing that what we attract may be even better than that![4]

Manage Stress and Tension

Tolerate the tension that naturally exists between your future vision and your present reality. Robert Fritz in *The Path of Least Resistance*[5] describes this tension as essential to the creative process that will eventually manifest your vision. He suggests that it is necessary to hold in your mind the simultaneous experiences of how you want your life to be and how your life actually is now. The gap between these two experiences will narrow in favor of the path that offers the least resistance. Managing the stress created by the tension between your present reality and your future vision is necessary to support your forward movement.

Be Patient

Don't expect your vision to occur immediately or to be crystal clear. Clarity will emerge over time as the experiences you have along the way shape and enhance the vision. It may take a while to arrive at your vision, as you review and revise it over the time it takes to get there. In truth, for those who learn to use this kind of visionary skill, arrival is a short-lived experience on the way to a continually evolving future always just tantalizingly out of reach. Your vision, like your life, is an ever-unfolding process, a journey over time, not necessarily a destination. Learning to relish the journey as much as the arrival is a useful way to manage the constant transitions and rapid changes prevalent today.

Reflect on Your Vision Frequently

Reflect frequently on the question "Where do you see yourself in the future? Doing what? With whom?" Consider starting a journal to capture and track the progressive development of your vision, using it as encouragement and motivation. Or carry a small notebook to capture fleeting thoughts or images related to your evolving vision. Often, when you turn your attention away from something you've been pondering, clarity emerges unexpectedly and spontaneously.

A Vision Exercise

Everyone has the capacity to visualize. The more you practice this ability, the stronger it will become. In some ways, visualizing is just another way of thinking, and you do it more often than you realize. To experience this, bring to mind your living room. Take about 15 seconds to recall the room and its contents, including any colors, associated sounds, or even aromas or physical sensations. Most likely you thought about your living room not in words but in images or, more specifically, in mental impressions of the locations of the furniture and objects of your living room. Perhaps you even had some associated sensory experiences, like the sound of birds outside your window. In bringing to mind your living room, you most likely imagined it, visualized it, saw it on the movie screen of your mind. In the same way, you can create images of your future and see yourself there. You can start by doing the exercise that follows.

Step 1: Begin by sitting quietly in a comfortable place where you won't be interrupted for about 30 minutes.

Step 2: Prepare yourself by practicing a breathing or relaxation exercise that quiets your mind, allows you to turn inward, and creates a receptive attitude within you.

Step 3: Reflect on the following questions and allow the answers to form as images or mental impressions on the movie screen of your mind rather than in words:

- What are you doing? With whom?
- In one year?
- In five years?
- In ten years?
- In any future time?
- What sounds, sensations, feelings arise?

Keep the emphasis on imagining yourself and what is going on around you and within you. Avoid developing a mental list of plans and tasks so that you can stimulate the right-brain creative process rather than left-brain problem solving.

Step 4: Answer the following questions and then use these answers to create your vision statement. Reflect on this frequently, pondering it over time and allowing it to shape and reshape itself.

- How I see myself in the future: ____________________
- What I am doing: ____________________
- Who I am with: ____________________
- Where I am and what is around me: ____________________
- What I hear and feel around me and within me: ____________________

WHAT DO YOU HAVE TO OFFER?

Now that you know a bit more about who you are, let's turn our attention to the second of the two components that determine your "product," namely what you have to offer. To know this, you need to be clear about what you are good at and what you prefer to spend most of your working time doing. Because there are so many nursing roles, you may find it difficult to determine what is best for you. An approach that can provide clarity is to understand how nursing roles blend specific work skills and activities with the core competencies that every nurse has. Even though nursing roles resist strict categorization, this approach provides a good enough general direction, which you can personalize and strengthen by combining the role with your mission, vision, and values/needs.

Nursing roles are extremely fluid; they are often influenced by the distinctive patient care needs in a particular setting. While each nurse is accountable to the standard of practice described in the Nurse Practice Act, to some degree the functions of the role are open to the interpretation of the nurse performing it. Nursing roles are also responsive to organizational policies, as well as to marketplace trends and changes. Hence, a nurse manager in one setting might work very differently from a nurse manager in another setting. Likewise, the job description for a medical-surgical direct care nurse will look different in a community hospital than in a major medical center.

Blending Basic Work Activities with Core Competencies in Nursing

A nursing role can be created by combining your preference for specific work activities with the core competencies necessary to perform them. Since basic work activities and core competencies are rarely performed in isolation from one another, the overlap that exists when describing them is reflective of the creative complexity inherent in nursing practice.

YOUR NURSING ROLE IS A BLENDING OF:				
Basic work skills	+	*Core nursing competencies*	=	*Your nursing role*
May include several categories of skills, with one or more in dominant use		May include more than one competency, with one or more being used primarily		Direct care nurse, or nurse manager, or staff development specialist, etc.

There are three generally recognized categories of work skills performed by the nurse. These are activities involving (1) people, (2) data and information, and (3) concepts and ideas. The box on page 159 specifies what comprises each of these three major categories.

In addition to work skills, there are five generally recognized core competencies inherent in the nursing role. These are (1) clinical, (2) managerial, (3) educational, (4) interpersonal, and (5) technical competencies. Each is described more fully below.

Clinical Competencies

These competencies describe the direct relationship a nurse has with a patient. They involve using specific technical skills within the nursing process of (1) assessing patient needs and responses, (2) planning the patient's care, (3) intervening with actions as required and necessary, and (4) evaluating the outcome of actions taken.

BASIC WORK SKILLS

People Skills	Data and Information Skills	Concept and Idea Skills
counseling	systematizing	creating
motivating	classifying information	translating
advocating	analyzing facts	visualizing
empathizing	compiling information	conceptualizing
coaching	summarizing	synthesizing
persuading	working with numbers	inventing
facilitating	testing hypothesis	designing
delegating	allocating resources	symbolizing
training	keeping records	acting
teaching	tabulating	innovating
listening	budgeting	extrapolating
advising	keeping inventories	demonstrating
interviewing	using logic	communicating
resolving conflicts	editing	evaluating
collaborating	mediating	presenting
providing	negotiating	reviewing
performing	informing	assisting
assessing	regulating	developing
appreciating	assigning	interpreting
intervening	appreciating	imagining
accomplishing	combining	affecting
alleviating	directing	affirming
defending	devising	confirming
enhancing	gathering	empowering
healing	generating	encouraging
improving	manifesting	fostering
nurturing	revising	illuminating
safeguarding	planning	involving
supporting	progressing	persuading
sustaining	validating	praising
touching		translating

The goal of the nurse employing these clinical competencies is to influence, support, or sustain a patient's physical, emotional, mental, spiritual, or interpersonal needs. All nurses who provide direct patient care utilize clinical competencies as well as the other four nursing competencies (described below). Likewise, many of the work activities related to people, data, and information, as well as concepts and ideas, are frequently represented in these clinical nursing competencies and are expressed in a variety of clinical nursing roles.

Examples of clinical competencies typically performed in the clinical role of the medical-surgical nurse at the novice or expert level might be these:

- Caring for postoperative patients
- Inserting IV lines
- Counseling families of dying patients
- Calculating medications
- Planning for discharge
- Teaching self-care to patients
- Interpreting data from monitor readouts
- Mentoring new nurses

Interpersonal Competencies

These competencies involve communicating with and relating to others. They often reflect—but are not limited to—the basic activities involved in people skills and concept and idea skills. Since clinical competencies cannot exist without interpersonal competencies, some of the examples listed above could just as easily be used here. Others include the following:

- Conducting medication teaching groups
- Empathizing with an anxious patient
- Collaborating with physicians
- Actively listening to a family member's concern
- Advocating for patients' rights
- Resolving conflicts between home health aides

Managerial Competencies

These competencies primarily involve planning, organizing, directing, and controlling system resources as well as the people in them. Data and information skills are often correlated with managerial competencies. General managerial competencies are part of the role of the nurse providing direct patient care as well as the nurse manager who oversees it. Here are some examples:

- Supervising nursing staff
- Conducting studies of sick time utilization
- Writing annual performance evaluations
- Writing handbooks for patient care technicians
- Using computers to develop budgets
- Designing new patient care delivery system
- Coordinating patient care activities
- Delegating responsibilities to others

Educational Competencies

These competencies primarily involve communicating concepts and ideas to others by means of explaining, teaching, and coaching. Once again, educational competencies are closely related to all the other nursing competencies, including, of course, interpersonal competencies. Examples include these:

- Teaching CPR to new mothers
- Teaching glucometer use to diabetic patients
- Designing nursing school curricula
- Creating orientation programs
- Mentoring new graduates
- Presenting online learning programs

Technical Competencies

These competencies involve the use of equipment and machinery, often complex and computerized, in correlation with other nursing competencies. Technical competencies rely heavily on the basic work abilities of data and information skills and cut across all nursing roles, in one way or another. Following are both high-tech and low-tech examples:

- Regulating ventilators
- Presenting online learning programs
- Taking blood pressures

- Hemodynamic monitoring
- Obtaining blood samples from central IV lines
- Using computers to input lab data
- Performing wound care
- Using computers to develop budgets

The Colors of Your Nursing Palette

Just as the primary colors of red, yellow, green, and blue form the basis of a vast color palette, so does the blending of these basic work skills with the core nursing competencies determine the "color" of your nursing practice palette. Nurses who prefer people skills make excellent direct care nurses at the novice or expert level as they develop the work skills that accompany this role. This role may vary among different workplaces and might include a higher or lower proportion of data and information skills or concept and idea skills. Likewise nurses with a high preference for data and information skills make good managers, and generally speaking, nurses with a high preference for concept and idea skills could make good nurse educators.

By blending these work skills and nursing competencies, you can create a career pathway to one or more of the clinical, administrative, educational, research, and consulting options in nursing practice and/or in the healthcare industry in general.

The box on the following page provides are more examples of nursing roles. Chapter 10: The Market Research Department of *You, Inc.* will elaborate on these roles and discuss the healthcare environments in which they can be found.

Levels of Nursing Proficiency

Something else to consider in describing your product is your current level of nursing proficiency. Pat Benner's classic and oft-quoted work *From Novice to Expert* is useful in making this self-assessment and ultimately helpful in determining whether this level of proficiency meets the requirements of your current or future employer. As discussed in chapter 5, Benner describes the five stages each nursing role has: the novice, advanced beginner, competent, proficient, and expert levels.

EXAMPLES OF NURSING ROLES CORRELATED WITH CORE COMPETENCIES AND BASIC WORK SKILLS

Clinical Competencies
Direct care nurse
Adult nurse practitioner
Psychiatric clinical nurse specialist
Community health nurse
Telephone triage nurse

Managerial Competencies
Nurse manager in a cardiac care center
Vice president, nursing and patient care services
Nurse researcher
Case manager

Educational Competencies
Staff development specialist
Professor, college of nursing
Community health educator
Childbirth educator

Interpersonal Competencies
Parish nurse
Bereavement counselor
Addictions and substance abuse specialist
Nurse psychotherapist

Technical Competencies
Informatics nurse
Critical care nurse
High-tech home care nurse
Sales representative for high-tech company

A novice has no experience and is typically a student nurse. The advanced beginner has limited, recurring experience. The level of competent describes a nurse who has at least two years of experience performing the same role. At the level Brenner identifies as proficient, the nurse can practice in situations requiring greater speed and flexibility, generally thought to occur after performing the role for three to five years. Nurses practicing at the expert level have achieved an intuitive and immediate level of mastery in complex situations that is thought to occur after a period of five or more years of experience in the same role. When you move between the generic roles of clinician, manager, or educator, you sometimes transition through these proficiency levels again, even as you bring transferable skills, abilities, and experiences along with you.

Take Karen, for example. An ANCC board-certified (at the generalist level) medical-surgical direct care nurse with ten years of experience in inpatient and ambulatory settings, she is practicing at the expert level according to Benner's model. She is also enrolled in an adult nurse practitioner program. When she graduates, she will be considered an advanced beginner in this new role and will need to give herself time to progress again through the levels of nursing practice proficiency. Intolerance of this necessary transition could affect Karen's professional self-esteem and career mobility.

Professional Certification

To be board certified at either the general practice level or at the specialist level announces to the healthcare marketplace your pride in meeting the high standards established by the nursing profession. Every business owner, including, of course, the nurse CEO of *You, Inc.,* would want to utilize this kind of product development and recognition.

The American Nurses Credentialing Center (ANCC), an arm of the American Nurses Association, offers board certification at the generalist and specialist levels in the following areas of nursing practice:

- Medicine and surgery
- Gerontology
- Pediatrics
- Perinatal, ob-gyn
- Community health
- Psychiatric/mental health

Certification in many nursing specialties is also available through other professional associations:

Nursing Specialty	**Professional Association**
Critical care nursing (CCRN)	American Association of Critical Care Nurses
Occupational health nursing (COHN)	American Board for Occupational Health Nurses
Emergency nursing (CEN)	Board of Certification for Emergency Nursing
Infection control nursing (CIC)	Certification Board of Infection Control

ANCC also offers the very prestigious Magnet status certification to healthcare organizations that have met certain standards of excellence. These Magnet status organizations have best practices that ensure quality patient care, as well as nursing practice environments that foster professional satisfaction. Some of the ways in which *You, Inc.* can take advantage of Magnet status include the following:

- Seek employment in Magnet status organizations.
- Identify your employment at a Magnet status facility on your resume.
- Find an appropriate way to mention this association in an interview.
- Determine if your present organization plans to apply for Magnet status. If not, consider lobbying for this or joining others who are doing so.
- Work on Magnet application committees in your organization. Be sure to include this on your resume.
- Network with nurses who work in Magnet status organizations, especially when you are considering seeking employment there.

CHAPTER 10

The Market Research Department of *You, Inc.*

> Any professional needs cross-cultural research and communication skills to be able to succeed in the future.
>
> —*Marye Tharp*

Of the many influences on the healthcare marketplace, the two most profound are the nursing shortage and the cost containment effects of managed care, resulting in truncated lengths of stay for patients in acute care hospitals followed by a continuation of care in an expanded landscape of healthcare facilities. This translates into a broadened continuum of care and an abundant and varied marketplace of enriched employment opportunities for the nurse CEO of *You, Inc.*

EMPLOYMENT TRENDS AND PREDICTIONS

The U.S. Department of Labor (*Occupational Outlook Handbook, 2010–11 Edition*[1]) identifies the trends and job outlook expected to affect registered nurse employment. A summary is presented below. Log on to *www.bls.gov/oco/print/ocos083.htm* for the full report which is updated annually.

Employment Trends

- Registered nurses represent the largest healthcare occupation, with 2.6 million jobs.
- About 60 percent of registered nurse jobs are in hospitals. The remaining jobs are elsewhere in the expanded healthcare marketplace.

- Employment of registered nurses is expected to grow 22 percent from 2008 to 2018, much faster than the average for all occupations. Growth will be driven by technological advances in patient care and an increased emphasis on preventative care.
- Employment of RNs will not grow at the same rate in all segments of the industry. The projected growth rate for RNs outside of the hospital is as follows:

Offices of physicians	48%
Home healthcare services	33%
Hospitals, public and private	17%
Employment services	24%
Nursing care facilities	25%

- About 581,500 new jobs are projected to be generated for registered nurses over the 2008–2018 period, one of the largest numbers among all occupations; overall job opportunities are expected to be excellent but may vary by employment setting.

Job Outlook

- Overall job opportunities are expected to be excellent for registered nurses because of the increased healthcare needs of the American people and the aging nursing workforce.
- Many qualified applicants are being turned away from nursing school because of a shortage of nursing faculty, which is expected to worsen. Many employers are relying on foreign-educated nurses to fill positions.
- Generally, RNs with at least a bachelor's degree will have better job propects. In addition, the four advanced practice specialties—clinical nurse specialists, nurse practitioners, nurse-midwives, and nurse-anesthetists—will be in high demand.
- More and more sophisticated procedures, as well as routine care once offered only in hospitals, are being performed in physician's offices, outpatient centers, and freestanding ambulatory surgical and emergency centers.
- To attract and retain qualified nurses, hospitals may offer sign-on bonuses, family-friendly work schedules, and subsidized training.
- A growing number of hospitals are experimenting with online bidding to fill open shifts for which nurses can volunteer to work

for premium wages. This may decrease the amount of mandatory overtime that nurses are all too often required to work.

Earnings

Median annual earnings of registered nurses were $63,750 in May 2009. The middle 50 percent earned between $52,520 and $77,970. The lowest 10 percent earned less than $43,970, and the highest 10 percent earned more than $93,700. For the latest national, state, and local earnings data, go to *www.bls.gov/OES/*.

THE HEALTHCARE MARKETPLACE

It is clear that the "hospitalcentric" age of healthcare, based on care during illness and injury, is ending. In its place has evolved a different framework that focuses on health as well as recovery from illness and injury. While hospitals traditionally took care of patients from admission to discharge, this new healthcare paradigm addresses the needs of people from birth to death.

This expanded environment represents a major change in healthcare delivery, with a shift from problem-oriented medical diagnosis and cure to a perspective on holism, prevention, and self-care. In this model, patients receive care along a pathway that spans the gamut between wellness and prevention of illness on one end to rehabilitation, long-term care, and end-of-life care on the other end, with nurses employed everywhere along the way. Vivien DeBack in "The New Practice Environment" in *Nurse Case Management in the 21st Century*[2] described the characteristics of this expanded healthcare system as follows:

- An emphasis on health, prevention, and wellness with an attention to risk factors, along with the expectation that people will take more responsibility for their health
- Intensive use of and reliance on information systems for patient documentation and for access to current practice information
- Reconsideration of human values with careful assessment of the balance between the expanding capability of technology and the need for humane treatment
- Focus on consumer and patient satisfaction with the encouragement of patient partnerships in decisions related to treatment
- Knowledge of treatment outcomes with emphasis on the most effective treatment under different conditions
- Constrained resources with cost containment to limit expenditures

- Coordination of resources with an emphasis on using teams to improve efficiency
- Growing awareness of the domestic and global healthcare issues of health, education, and public safety

EMPLOYMENT OPTIONS IN THE HEALTHCARE MARKETPLACE

In the expanding healthcare marketplace, nurses will find interesting and satisfying employment opportunities. Use the examples below to help find the best match for your product—your nursing skills and competencies.

Acute Care Hospitals

This is among the most familiar of the facilities along the continuum of care. This is where most people expect to go when ill or injured and where the majority of nurses will continue to work, but nurses will work here differently than did previous generations. Nurses in this extremely fluid, high-tech environment will see fast-paced action, rapid turnover of acutely or critically ill patients, and short-term relationships with patients who will continue recovering in the post–acute care facilities described below.

Transitional Hospitals

These facilities continue the care for patients who are still acutely ill but are in stable condition. The patients in these facilities require intensive, skilled care from a wide variety of healthcare disciplines and have an average minimum stay of around 25 days. For example, following his horseback riding accident, the actor Christopher Reeve was cared for in a transitional hospital after he was stabilized in an acute care hospital.

Because the transitional hospital doesn't have to fund services typically found in acute care hospitals, such as ambulatory clinics and emergency departments, it can provide a broad range of interventions, including ICU-type services, at about one-third to one-half the cost of acute care hospitals. This, of course, makes transitional hospitals quite attractive to managed-care companies. Rather than duplicate such services as lab and X-ray, they may purchase them when needed from affiliated agencies, thereby avoiding the costly purchase and maintenance of these services. This is a great practice environment for the nurse who enjoys high-tech, acute/critical care but wants a longer-term relationship with patients and enjoys a strong emphasis on teaching and patient self-care.

Sub-acute Care Facilities

The patient requiring care in sub-acute facilities falls somewhere between needing less intensive care than an acute care hospital would provide but more than what the long-term facility can offer. This, along with rehabilitation, makes for a unique combination of services. The care provided is short-term (average length of stay is 5 to 14 days) with a focused plan geared to helping the patient achieve a specific goal (for example, walking independently with a cane following hip replacement surgery). The patient is referred to the next level of care when ready. These patients are stable but can still be quite ill, often requiring high-tech monitoring. As in the transitional hospital, they receive skilled interventions from a multidisciplinary team. Nurses in this type of facility will find themselves developing specialties such as, for example, orthopedic nursing.

Long-Term Care Facilities

The change in name from *nursing home* to *long-term care facility* reflects the influence of changing economics and reimbursement mechanisms. These facilities restructured their services in response to the need to provide a higher level of skilled intervention for their patients when they became ill, rather than transferring them to more costly facilities like acute care hospitals. In addition to being the extension of the patient's family and community that it has always been, the long-term care facility now has an increasing number of specialty units, all designed to treat the patient while ill. Examples include dementia and AIDS care.

Hospice Services

Many hospice services are part of and/or administered by home care programs or by inpatient facilities, such as acute care hospitals, in collaboration with the home care agency's visiting nurses. Hospice care provides services and support to terminally ill patients (generally with a prognosis of six months or less to live), including skilled nursing care, home health aides and attendants, and specialized medical equipment as indicated. The combined focus on physical care and emotional support is often described by hospice nurses as both rewarding and challenging.

Assisted Living Facilities

This mostly privately funded option provides several levels of healthcare and personal care services for the elderly who are well and want to live independently, as well as special facilities for the frail elderly. This level of care may be available to the physically and emotionally disabled as well. Assisted living facilities offer apartment-style living along with such personal support as dining room meals served in an attractive, restaurant-like atmosphere, household cleaning, and recreational activities. The residents enjoy the benefits of security, companionship, and access to ongoing healthcare or, if necessary, emergency care. Ambulatory or inpatient care, when needed, is provided through a network of affiliated agencies. Even patients with dementia and Alzheimer's disease can be accommodated in the specialized units of some assisted living facilities.

Home Healthcare Services

Technological advances, as well as economic restraints, have fostered a boom in home healthcare services. This is believed to be the fastest-growing segment of the healthcare marketplace, with high-tech home care and psychiatric home care growing the fastest. Today's home care patient tends to be more severely or chronically ill than ever before. Home care agencies fall into three general categories: licensed, certified, and long-term.

- Licensed agencies provide private-duty nursing as well as assistive and personal care support, often from home health attendants.
- Certified agencies care for sicker patients, often those discharged "sicker and quicker" from acute care hospitals, and offer a broad range of services, such as rehabilitation, assistance in daily living activities from home health aides, and social service support.
- Long-term home care agencies provide supportive care to those patients who are chronically ill and qualify for a long-term, inpatient care facility but who choose to remain at home.

Adult Day Care Services

These facilities provide skilled nursing, assisted personal care, and long-term care to patients who may or may not be receiving simultaneous home care services. Patients come to day care for socialization or for such skilled nursing services as insulin monitoring and tracheostomy care. These facilities provide the patients with an enhanced quality of life and the caregiver relative with an excellent option for rest and relief or just the freedom to do errands or go to work.

Community-Based Services

These familiar healthcare facilities have long existed in the community outside the traditional walls of acute care hospitals. These services include the following:

- Ambulatory healthcare centers, including physician or nurse-based practices, freestanding or hospital-based clinics, and health maintenance organizations for all healthcare specialties, including mental health and substance abuse
- Ambulatory surgical centers
- Occupational and corporate healthcare services and wellness programs found in most traditional workplaces as well as more exotic locations, like movie sets, circuses, sporting events, concerts, resorts, camps, spas, health clubs, and weight loss centers
- Family planning centers
- Birthing centers
- Pain management centers
- Wound care centers
- Hemodialysis centers
- Outreach centers of churches, synagogues, and other religious institutions
- Forensic and prison healthcare services and facilities
- School health offices and centers
- Shelters, housing assistance, and mobile crisis programs for the homeless and mentally ill

Supporting and/or Affiliating Services

These for-profit and nonprofit services form a web of support that serves and/or affiliates with healthcare organizations of all types, including institutions for the education of healthcare personnel. Their services include these:

- **Pharmaceutical and medical supply companies:** These companies hire nurses to market their products to a variety of healthcare organizations and agencies. Competencies required might include teaching skills. Knowledge of the product is expected. An example is experience in the use of specialized dressings for wound care.
- **Healthcare consulting organizations:** These include a vast array of services and programs, including computer consulting, organizational redesign experts, healthcare accrediting organizations, and so on.

- **Personnel supply agencies:** These provide professional and ancillary staff to healthcare organizations.
- **Schools and colleges:** These educate nurses and other healthcare personnel.

NURSING ROLES IN THE HEALTHCARE MARKETPLACE

Now that you are armed with a map of healthcare's territories, you can consider the nursing roles and employment options associated with them. As healthcare continues to evolve and restructure its services along the continuum of care, nursing roles and responsibilities will evolve as well.

The three generic roles of direct care nurse, nurse-manager, and nurse-educator, at the basic or advanced levels of practice, can be found in a variety of employment venues.

In the chart below, these generic nursing roles are combined with examples of nursing practice options and potential places of employment along the continuum of care. This is not an all-inclusive list but does represent a way to think about the employment opportunities available to you. Consider reading profiles of nurses in these roles online or in print publications like *Nursing Spectrum*. This will allow you a glimpse into what life as a nurse is like in a role of interest to you.

GENERIC NURSING ROLE	EXAMPLE OF NURSING PRACTICE OPTION	POTENTIAL PLACE OF EMPLOYMENT ALONG THE CONTINUUM OF CARE
Manager Educator	Informatics nurse	All settings
Educator	Nursing school faculty	Colleges and schools of nursing Continuing education sites
Manager or Direct care nurse	Case manager	Inpatient settings

GENERIC NURSING ROLE	EXAMPLE OF NURSING PRACTICE OPTION	POTENTIAL PLACE OF EMPLOYMENT ALONG THE CONTINUUM OF CARE
Direct care nurse	Risk alert manager	Community settings
Direct care nurse	Utilization review nurse	Health insurance companies
Direct care nurse	Telephone triage nurse	Managed care companies
		Insurance companies
		Hospital EDs
Direct care nurse	Telephone triage nurse	Health insurance companies
Direct care nurse Manager Educator	Infection control nurse	Private and government agencies of homeland security for protection against bioterrorism attacks
Direct care nurse Manager Educator	Infection control nurse	Many inpatient and outpatient settings
Direct care nurse Educator	Nurse consultant	Pharmaceutical companies
		Hospital supply companies
		Private practice
Manager	Legal nurse consultant	Attorney's office
Educator	Paralegal nurse	Risk management departments in all settings

GENERIC NURSING ROLE	EXAMPLE OF NURSING PRACTICE OPTION	POTENTIAL PLACE OF EMPLOYMENT ALONG THE CONTINUUM OF CARE
Educator Direct care nurse	Paralegal nurse	Risk management in all settings
Direct care nurse Manager	Nurse entrepreneur	Private practice in psychotherapy
Manager Administrator	Nurse entrepreneur	Owner of home care agency
Direct care nurse Educator	Advance practice nurse	Nurse-run clinic
Direct care nurse	Nurse practitioner	Nurse-physician group Practice
Direct care nurse	Clinical nurse specialist	Multiple inpatient and outpatient settings

STRATEGIES FOR SUCCESS

Take your role as the nurse CEO of *You, Inc.* seriously. Develop a self-employed attitude, managing your career as if it were your own business and attending to all the departments of *You, Inc.* in ways that keep it aligned with the best employment options possible.

Recognize the need to develop the following nursing competencies, knowing that they will be increasingly emphasized in the models of healthcare emerging in the 21st century:

- Advocacy for patients accessing healthcare services
- Teaching, learning, and coaching
- Resource management
- Critical thinking and problem solving
- Flexibility in thinking and acting
- Relationship and communication skills for collaborative team practice

- Information management skills
- Willingness to learn and utilize technology
- Keen sensitivity to and support of cultural diversity
- Community health and systems perspectives

Work towards preserving a front row seat in the theater of healthcare employment. This includes having the following:

- Bachelor of Science in Nursing
- Professional certification at the generalist or specialist level
- Current and relevant continuing education
- Broad cross-training
- Superb self-care
- Comfort with technology

Be flexible. Be prepared to move to what's new and what's next. Be a trend watcher. Take the advice of futurists and forecasters seriously when they say that a change affecting the way you live and work will occur every six months.

See the opportunities and challenges, rather than danger or threats, in new work opportunities that come your way, whether expected or unexpected. Manage the stress of change that often accompanies something new.

Revise, revise, and revise again. Keep the root of the word *revise* in mind. It means "to see and to see again; to look over something; to correct or improve; to make a new version of; to take another look; to update." Revise and update your mission, your vision, your resume, and your nursing skills and competencies in alignment with current and emerging trends in the healthcare marketplace.

Stay ahead of your technological learning curve. Nurses everywhere along the continuum of care can no longer get by without some level of comfort with healthcare technology as well as at least a beginning level of computer literacy and Internet use. While you may be able to choose low-tech versus high-tech care, there is no longer any such thing as "no-tech."

Unless you are interested in the fast-paced, high-tech environment of acute care hospitals where relationships with patients are short-term, seek employment elsewhere among the vast opportunities along the continuum of care.

Seek out employers who are aware of the need to restructure roles and staffing patterns, as well as the need to improve working conditions, to attract and retain nurses. This is especially true of the mature nurse. Since all nurses will benefit from the workplace accommodations aimed at mature nurses, even if you are not a mature nurse, seek out those employers for yourself as well.

Take self-care seriously to ensure that you have the resilience and stamina needed to manage the demands of this profession and to prevent burnout and compassion fatigue.

KEEPING CURRENT

To obtain the most up-to-date information about the healthcare marketplace, access the websites and homepages of professional associations and organizations, as well as government bureaus and agencies. Here are some suggestions:

- **Professional and government organizations:**
  - U.S. Department of Labor: *www.dol.gov*
  - Bureau of Labor Statistics: *www.bls.gov*
  - National League for Nursing: *www.nln.org*
  - American Association of Colleges of Nursing: *www.aacn.nche.edu*
  - American Nurses Association: *www.nursingworld.org*
- **Online nursing networks and career information sites:**
  - *nursing.advanceweb.com*
  - *www.nurse.com*
  - *www.monster.com*
  - *www.careerbuilder.com*
  - *www.nursingworld.com*

CHAPTER 11

The Strategic Planning Department of *You, Inc.*

Like all successful business owners, the nurse CEO of *You, Inc.* knows that a well-developed strategic plan is essential to success. Your strategic plan puts a foundation under your vision and translates your mission as a nurse into reality. Your goals and their accompanying tasks become the pathway upon which you travel towards achieving what you once only dreamed or imagined. A well-thought-out marketing plan reflects the special attributes of the work you do and helps you identify where to find the best match for your product (your nursing skills and competencies) in the healthcare marketplace. It takes the ideas and data generated from the other departments of *You, Inc.* and pulls them together into a coherent whole. Planning creates clarity and focus, essential for guiding yourself through multiple and varied employment options.

Your strategic plan is a road map, a time schedule, and a feedback mechanism all rolled into one. Combine this plan with your commitment to succeed and the support of people in your professional and personal networks, and you have the ingredients for excellent career mobility and success.

To develop your strategic plan, follow the steps in this chapter. Reflect on each section as it relates to your current or anticipated employment goals. Revisit and revise your plan periodically. You should validate the marketability of your plan about every six months, since futurists and forecasters predict that changes affecting your work or personal life may occur that frequently.

STEP 1: DESCRIBE YOUR MISSION, YOUR VISION, AND YOUR VALUES

Your mission, vision, and values describe who you are as a nurse and what you have to offer an employer. Together they represent what will give you career satisfaction and sustain you through the winds of change by grounding you in what is most meaningful and important to you, personally and professionally. Refer to your answers and reflections to the exercises in chapter 9 and fill in the blanks below:

My mission (what I do):

____________________, ______________________, and __________________

(Your three verbs from Step 1)

My values or principles (what I stand for):

____

(Your core values or principles from Step 2)

To or for, among or with (whom you help):

____

(The group or cause from Step 3)

My mission statement is:

____

____

____

My vision of myself as a nurse:

____

My professional and personal values:

____

____

____

STEP 2: IDENTIFY YOUR BUSINESS/NURSING ROLE

As discussed in chapter 8, the name of your business is *You, Inc.* This is your self-owned nursing practice, and you are the chief executive officer. Your nursing business provides a product/service expressed in the role you perform. This role is a blending of basic work skills and core nursing competencies. Refer to how you identified your nursing role in chapter 9 and then work through the steps below to describe the product you currently have to offer employers.

Basic work skills:

1. Reflect on your present job or one you may be considering.
2. List all the work skills and activities that this job requires.

____

3. Which skills and activities do you

   like doing? ______________________________

   dislike doing?______________________________

   want to do more of?__________________________

4. Refer to the general categories of basic work skills below. Which do you prefer to spend the most time doing? Rank them in your order of preference, with 1 signifying most preferred and 3 signifying least preferred:

   _____ People skills

   _____ Data and information skills

   _____ Concept and idea skills

Core nursing competencies:

1. Refer to the discussion of core nursing competencies in chapter 9 and the list below.

2. Which do you prefer to spend the most time doing? Rank these in your order of preference, with 1 signifying most preferred and 3 signifying least preferred:

_____ Clinical competencies

_____ Managerial competencies

_____ Educational competencies

_____ Interpersonal competencies

_____ Technical competencies

Your business/nursing role: Review and summarize your responses to the questions above and then fill in the following blanks:

The nursing business you are currently in is: ______________________________

An example of this role is: ____

Healthcare employers interested in this nursing role/business are:

____

____

STEP 3: ASSESS YOUR LEVEL OF NURSING PRACTICE PROFICIENCY

Using Benner's model of nursing proficiency[1] as described in chapter 5 and again in chapter 9, identify the level of proficiency you have now or the level that's expected in the role you are considering. Use this assessment as a way to match your qualifications to employer expectations.

❒ Level I = Novice

❒ Level II = Advanced Beginner

- ❒ Level III = Competent
- ❒ Level IV = Proficient
- ❒ Level V = Expert

STEP 4: SELECT A HEALTHCARE TERRITORY

Identify an employment option you would like to target by analyzing and reviewing the traditional and emerging territories along the continuum of care discussed in chapter 10.

Select the geographical location most attractive to you, as well as those locations that most likely contain your target market. Determine what employment trends or predictions might affect your choice. For example, if your specialty is psychiatry and mental health, you might want to target health services for Iraqi veterans suffering from posttraumatic stress disorder. This is a fast-growing, emerging segment of the healthcare marketplace.

Identify your customer. Which employer is most likely to want what you have to offer? For example, the new BSN graduate who wants to work in critical care but has no experience will find customers/employers in acute care hospitals that have their own on-site critical care training programs in which they develop the staff they can't find elsewhere during this nursing shortage. Complete the following:

Your target market is: ____

Your customer is: ____

Related societal and cultural trends are: ______________________________

____

Related employment trends are: ____________________________________

____

Qualifications for this target market are: _____________________________

____

Are you currently qualified?

- ❐ Yes
- ❐ No
- ❐ Perhaps, if . . .

If you answered no or perhaps, select another option or develop a plan to improve your qualifications for this position; see Step 6.

STEP 5: KNOW HOW TO STAND OUT!

No business owner who intends to succeed would ever think of investing time, money, and other resources in a service or product without an awareness of who else was also offering it and how their business matched up against the competition. Neither should you! The way to keep your career satisfying and invigorating is to stand out so you don't fade out.

Answer the following questions:

How is your product/service (your nursing skills and competencies) as good as or better than that of others who have the same or similar skills and competencies? Consider your experience, credentials, ongoing continuing education, professional certification, etc. These will be important selling features in job interviews.

____

____

If you and five other nurses applied for a job you wanted, what would make you at least as qualified or even more qualified? How would you stand out? Consider transferable skills, interpersonal style, communications skills, personal interests, etc.

____

____

What skills, competencies, experiences, or ideas can you identify that would contribute to and potentially improve the quality of service for the organization in which you are considering employment? Think beyond the minimum expectation of showing up for work and performing the tasks required in your job description. Consider committees you have served on, interests you have such as diabetic teaching using Internet resources, etc. List these here:

____

____

____

Below are professional and personal characteristics employers are likely to expect. The more of these you possess, the more you will stand out from others. Identify the ones you already have or are in the process of developing.

Professional experience:

_____ Has targeted, progressive, cumulative work as a generalist and/or specialist.

_____ Has examples of work experiences that contributed value to the workplace.

_____ Is aware of, is able to support, and can contribute to patient-focused care in a consumer-oriented business environment.

_____ Has diverse, transferable skills.

_____ Has participated in cross-training.

_____ Has completed continuing education.

_____ Is computer literate and Internet savvy.

_____ Has a Bachelor of Science in Nursing.

_____ Has advanced educational preparation commensurate with career goals.

_____ Has ANCC board certification as a generalist or specialist (or other professional certification).

_____ Has professional membership(s).

_____ Additional: ________________________________

Personal characteristics:

_____ Is flexible, adaptive, assertive, confident, empowered.

_____ Is self-directed and team-savvy.

_____ Is an innovative problem solver.

_____ Does not accept status quo.

_____ Is willing to take risks.

_____ Learns from mistakes.

_____ Possesses conflict resolution skills.

_____ Is a critical thinker.

_____ Is a master networker.

_____ Additional: ________________________________

Note: This is by no means a complete list. Add to this list; personalize it to your situation.

How Well Do You Stand Out?

Based on your answers in Step 5, use the following scale to rate your ability to stand out and compete effectively for employment opportunities:

- ❒ 1 = unable to compete effectively
- ❒ 2 = need work to compete effectively
- ❒ 3 = able to compete under some circumstances
- ❒ 4 = able to compete in most circumstances
- ❒ 5 = able to compete effectively

STEP 6: IDENTIFY NEEDS AND RESOURCES

Now you are ready to identify specifically your professional, personal, and interpersonal skills, resources, strengths, and abilities. Fill in the blanks on the pages that follow.

Your needs and resources:

Current, transferable skills (include nonnursing work):

____

____

Professional and personal strengths and weaknesses (selling points and areas needing improvement):

____

____

Professional and personal priorities (consider personal and professional situations):

____

Inner obstacles (limiting beliefs such as "I'm too old, too young, too busy, etc."):

____

____

Outer obstacles (such as lack of experience or credentials):

____

____

Training and education needs:

____

____

Insurance, licensure, certification needs and issues:

____

____

Networking needs (see chapter 12):

____

____

Professional network (list key names):

____

____

Personal network (list key names):

____

____

Networking activities and events to target for attending (include online social networking sites):

____

____

Financial needs and issues:

____

____

Stress management and self-care needs:

____

____

Career guidance needed:

____

____

Additional needs and considerations:

____

____

What is the status of your advertising and sales tools, which include your resume, your interview skills, professional portfolio, and business card? Your resume is your means of advertising, and the interview is where you have the opportunity to sell your nursing product. These tools will be discussed in depth in chapters 13 and 14. Check the box below that best describes the status of these important career tools:

Advertising tools/resume:

- ❒ Nonexistent
- ❒ Needs revision
- ❒ Updated and ready

Sales tools/interview skills:

- ❒ Nonexistent
- ❒ Needs revision
- ❒ Updated and ready

Professional portfolio:

- ❒ Nonexistent
- ❒ Needs revision
- ❒ Updated and ready

Business card:

- ❒ Nonexistent
- ❒ Needs revision
- ❒ Updated and ready

STEP 7: DETERMINE YOUR RISK POTENTIAL AND RISK TOLERANCE

Risk is a relative term. It is an integral part of life and a familiar companion to all successful business owners, including you, the nurse CEO of *You, Inc.* To take a risk means to experience the unfamiliar, which is typically accompanied by a degree of stress and anxiety, a natural human response to potentially destabilizing circumstances. Without some degree of risk and uncertainty in our lives, we could never grow, either personally or professionally.

We intuitively know this as children, but many of us lose this confidence as adults, sometimes adopting the limiting beliefs of others. A baby unable to risk falling might never stand or walk. And, of course, only through falling many times can the baby finally learn to walk. And, so it is with learning throughout our lives, unless we let limiting beliefs stop us.

An example of a limiting belief is "If I fail, I will look stupid and be embarrassed." How different this person might feel if that belief was replaced by something like "Failure is nothing more than data pointing to what needs to be done differently to accomplish my goal." Henry Ford captured this well when he said, "Whether you believe you can or you can't, you are right."

Clearly, all risks are not equal. Investing in a pyramid scheme or lending someone more money who has not repaid what was already borrowed are examples of risks not worth taking. Other risks might have a good or even great possibility of a beneficial outcome, but even these are not guaranteed to succeed with certainty. These intelligent, or informed, risks are the ones that are essential for career and personal success. In fact, there could be more negative consequences than positive ones if we are so risk-averse that we reject informed risk too often.

A good marketing plan provides you with the information you need to take career risks with the greatest degree of security possible. Because the future cannot be predicted, no one can say with certainty that this or that risk will be worth taking. However, if you believe that every experience is an opportunity to learn something, even if the risk does not pay off in the way you imagined, you will still have gained more than you lost. Not being able to see the future should not fully stop us from moving into it in a way that is as informed as possible.

To determine your tolerance for the risk associated with the career step you are considering, complete the risk-safety assessment below and interpret your score according to the scale that follows.

Risk-Safety Assessment

Read each statement below and rate it by placing a number in the space that precedes the statement according to the following scale:

- 1 = very safe — 5 = more risky than safe
- 2 = mostly safe — 6 = somewhat risky
- 3 = somewhat safe — 7 = mostly risky
- 4 = more safe than risky — 8 = very risky

_____ Personal or professional financial costs

_____ Influence of career goal on other priorities

_____ Ability to manage the stress of change and uncertainty

_____ Relative stability of the healthcare market segment you are targeting

_____ Additional personal or professional considerations:

____

To interpret your score, total the points in the columns above:

Low risk = 5 to 12 points

Moderate risk = 13 to 28 points

High risk = 29 to 40 points

Is this career goal feasible?

❒ Yes

❒ No (rethink what you need to do)

❒ Perhaps, if I ______________________________

Profit and Loss Analysis

This term is used by business owners to denote a method of assessing overall financial risk. Here, it is translated to mean the overall risk of your next career step summarized in pros and cons. Use the data from your risk analysis above, as well as answers to other questions in this section, to identify how much there may be to gain or to lose:

Pros of pursuing this career goal (reasons to pursue): ___________________

____

Cons of pursuing this career goal (reasons not to pursue): _______________

____

What I might profit or gain from taking this career step is:

____

What I might lose is: ____

____

STEP 8: CREATE A PLAN FOR THIS CAREER STEP

This next step brings together everything you have discovered in this section. Begin by stating a clear goal in specific and concrete terms. The more specific you are, the easier your goal will be to implement. Use action verbs and outcomes that can be measured or seen.

For example, "I will find a job as a nurse," is vague and not easily measured. An example of a goal that is stated in a more useful way for tracking your progress is "Within two months, I will find a job as a medical-surgical nurse in an acute care hospital that has at least 500 beds and an orientation program of at least two weeks."

Attach to your goal the tasks you need to do to achieve it. An example might include updating your resume or preparing for the interview. Make the tasks as specific as possible, breaking it into its smallest components. Examples of tasks required to write or revise your resume might include finding your old resume, talking to colleagues about their resumes, or making an appointment with a resume writer. Each task should have a target date of completion to keep you on track.

It is often necessary to revise your goals. This may not be evident until action is taken and you have an opportunity to evaluate the results. Tracking your experience and progress helps you make the revisions that are essential to achieving your goal. For example, as you move along, it may become clear that the goal of finding a new job is mistimed and needs to be delayed for a while. Or you may discover that the target dates were too ambitious and, while the goal is still feasible, you need to make adjustments to the task list and time line.

Use the outline below to organize the goals and tasks required to achieve this next career step.

GOALS AND TASKS

My goal is: ____

Tasks (What actions are needed?):

____

Target dates (by when?):

____

Outcomes (Evaluate the results and identify what's next):

____

Revisions (Develop new goals and/or tasks as needed):

____

STEP 9: JOB SEARCH STRATEGIES

Now that you have your plan, it's time to determine where to take it, who might be interested, and who your customer is.

The more time you are willing to devote to your job search, the more it will pay off for you. There is more to finding a new job than sending out a resume and then sitting back, waiting for the phone to ring. Some tips to keep you on track are the following:

- Keep track of your progress, in writing, by using the marketing plan you completed in this chapter.
- Set aside scheduled time each day to track your progress.

- Create a space in your home to keep related supplies and information. Consider including some motivational or inspirational material in the form of quotes, pictures, or symbols to encourage you. Here's one: "Faith is the daring of the soul to go farther than it can see" (William Newton Clarke).
- Get organized. Start a folder or develop a filing system for each employer contact you have made and note the time of the contact, the result of the contact, the next scheduled contact, your impressions of the conversation, and next steps.
- Think carefully before sending out resumes and query letters to potential employers who may not be looking for what you have to offer. A "shotgun" approach can succeed in certain circumstances, but it can also disperse your energy, especially if time is short. Each letter you send requires follow-up contact of some sort, making this a very time-intensive way to search for a job. On the other hand, the payoff could be big if you are seeking a job that is not often advertised or is otherwise hard to find.
- Tell everyone in your professional and personal network (online and in person) what kind of job you are seeking.
- Use the job postings within your present organization to generate leads and possibilities; ask your peers and colleagues in other organizations to do likewise for you.
- Attend career fairs, including online virtual job fairs and other similar events. Don't forget your resume and business card. Be sure to dress professionally, and expect to be interviewed by potential employers.
- Peruse healthcare and nursing-specific classified ads in newspapers and nursing publications, such as *Advance for Nurses* and *Nursing Spectrum*. It is a good idea to track job openings even if you are not considering making a move. This is an excellent way to monitor trends in the current marketplace and keep your qualifications aligned with what employers are seeking.
- Use the Internet for employment information and job listings. Most healthcare organizations and institutions have homepages that not only describe them but have job postings as well. Examples of nursing specific career sites with job postings are these:
    - *www.monster.com*
    - *www.nurse.com*
    - *nursing.advanceweb.com*
    - *www.nursingworld.com*

CHAPTER 12

The Networking Department of *You, Inc.*

Networks are loose, dynamic webs of personal and professional alliances, forged for the purpose of obtaining knowledge, exchanging information, and sharing support. Networks are everywhere people are, both online and in person.

Networks can emerge spontaneously or be created intentionally. You can take them with you, leave them behind, form new ones, create formal or informal ones, merge old and new networks, or link your network with the networks of others. Professional networks are essential to encouraging your vision, strengthening your mission, and validating your values/needs, the three important components of your nursing product/service, all of which are necessary to ensuring career stability and professional satisfaction, especially during times of change.

In this age of information, the currency of exchange is knowledge and information. The relationships in networks provide a way to obtain and utilize this currency, exchange it with others, and make it grow. Participating in networks is a way to invest in yourself and in *You, Inc.*, which is as important as any financial investment you could ever make. Because registered nurses are knowledge workers, networks become essential links to and repositories for the vast amount of ever-increasing information that you alone could never completely acquire or keep current enough. Successful nurses know how to access the information they need, often rather quickly, from online networks and Internet portals, as well as from the many traditional in-person networks they keep active. Networks are information and knowledge storehouses waiting for a time when you need what's in them.

Part of the satisfaction of participating in networks is the opportunity to give to others, as well as to receive from them. It can feel as good to respond supportively to a message posted online by a despairing new graduate as to support this new graduate in person. The process of helping this new nurse provides you with an opportunity to see and benefit from your own growth and experience and to realize how far you have come. Getting through challenges is always easier with support and mentoring, a good deal of which is done in networks.

A NETWORK IN ACTION

A network represents the connections between and among people; some have direct relationships to each other, while others are like distant relatives who are once or twice removed. You may not know the person who has the information you need, but in a large enough network, you are only "one or two degrees of separation" from obtaining it. Consider how the nurse in the following example makes use of networks.

> Joan, a medical-surgical nurse with a BSN and four years of experience in an oncology unit, is about to enter a master's program. She is also considering becoming board certified in oncology nursing. She wonders if certification would really benefit her professionally and is concerned about whether she will be able to engage in the certification process and begin school at the same time.
>
> She asks three people she works with, Tom, Mary, and Barbara, as well as Judy, a nurse in one of her social-networking groups, what they know about it and if they think doing both is a good idea. As you can see from figure 12.1, Joan got the information she needed through direct and indirect links. She only communicated directly with Tom, Mary, Barbara, and Judy, who each had information acquired from people Joan did not know: Jill, Bob, Richard, and Marie. And the information about certification that these four people supplied came from another four people also unknown to Joan.
>
> Joan got the information she needed and more by extending her reach beyond those people with whom she had direct contact. When she found out that the certification exam would be given again next year, she felt less pressured about studying for it at the same time as beginning school.

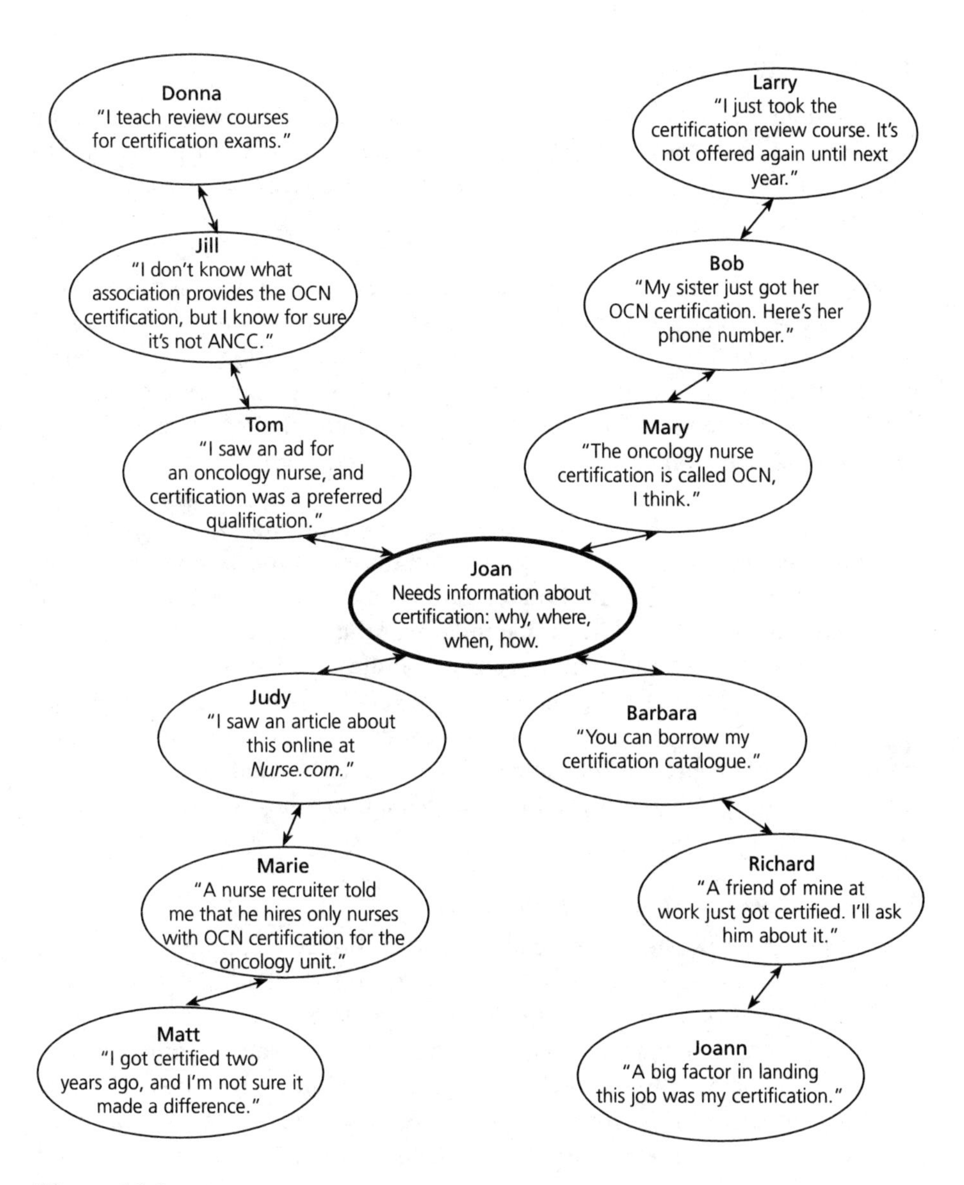

Figure 12.1

NETWORKING ONLINE

Personal and professional networking has moved to cyberspace, where a wide variety of websites bring people together via the Internet. The following are descriptions of online networking experiences in which you can participate professionally, personally, or both.

Online Social Networking

Like millions of people across a broad demographic, nurses are making use of online social networks (broadly called *social media*) to participate in communities in which information can be obtained, concerns shared, and ideas explored.

Social networks linking friends and classmates began appearing on the Internet around 2004. Today, the most well-known and heavily trafficked social networks include Facebook, Twitter, LinkedIn, and YouTube. The popularity and indispensability of these networking tools cannot be overemphasized. For example, LinkedIn, a business- and career-oriented site, currently claims 20 million users in 150 countries.

In 2009, Nicholoson Kovac, a marketing communications agency (*www.nicholsonkovac.com*), conducted a study about the use of social media by nurses and physicians. The results indicated that nurses and physicians were about a year behind the general public in making use of this means of communicating and accessing information. The results also indicated that 87 percent of the nurses used the Internet for professional reasons, 77 percent used Facebook, 25 percent used LinkedIn, and only 11 percent used Twitter. Among the nurses in the survey who were not yet using social media, 65 percent planned to do so in the near future. Where do you find yourself among these data?

ANANurseSpace (www.nursingworld.org)

This is the American Nurses Association's (ANA) protected online professional networking site designed exclusively for nurses and student nurses. Here you will find facilitators or bloggers (short for "web loggers") who start dialogues by posting a topic of interest that sometimes becomes an ongoing journal. Everyone who belongs to the site can respond. In addition to choosing one of the many nursing communities within ANANurseSpace to which you want to belong, you can create a profile that identifies you and helps you build professional contacts. The following box contains ANA President Rebecca M. Patton's inaugural blog for ANANurseSpace.

ANA President Rebecca M. Patton's Inaugural Blog for ANANurseSpace

Greetings Friends and Fellow Nurses:

Welcome to the first Inaugural "ANA President's Blog." Yes, with the help of my 9- and 12-year-old nephews, I am jumping into blogging. Their expertise and lack of inhibition have motivated my desire to start this regular "ANA President's Blog." So I am all ears to any tips you might have.

The ANA President's Blog will occur every two weeks. I will be posting my blog typically on the 1st and 15th of each month. I look forward to and suspect your responses will be invaluable in many of the discussions that will occur.

I am certain some of the blogging will be spirited. Within ANA, we respect the diversity of our membership and we are all better for it. As you may know, free-flowing and broad-based debate and discussion is a mainstay among the Association's national membership. Clearly, we share a deep and abiding love of and respect for nursing as it is meant to be practiced; a sincere determination to accomplish those changes that make a difference for our profession and our patients; and a shared respect for our knowledge, skills and abilities. This is more than a common ground upon which to build an agenda, it is what bonds us and defines us as one single profession.

So let's jump into one of the spirited discussions as the first ANA President's Blog.

Which ratio do you want to have for staffing your unit? One mandated by your legislator who knows nothing about the particulars of your unit or one determined by a staffing committee of staff nurses and managers that have access to your unique work situation?

Safe Staffing Saves Lives (*www.safestaffingsaveslives.org*) representing ANA's interest in this issue is so strong that we have made it a centerpiece of our decades-long effort on behalf of health system reform. We believe the proper ratio depends on the circumstances at a given hospital or other care setting. It requires principles that should include factors such as each unit's patient acuity, skill mix and experience of the staff, available support services for staff, and available technology.

What do you think? And most importantly, how do we get there?

Thanks in advance for your response.

Do you have a response to this question about staffing ratios? Log on to ANA's website (*www.nursingworld.org*) and click on ANANurseSpace if you want to join the conversation or read responses to this blog.

LinkedIn (www.linkedin.com)

This is one of the most well-known sites in which you need to be introduced by a "link"—a person whom you know. Then you build your network by inviting people you know to become linked to you. If they agree, you then have access to their networks as well.

Employment recruiters sometimes use LinkedIn and other social-networking sites as recruitment tools, especially in tight labor markets such as nursing. Consider whether or not you want this type of access to your professional information. Craft your profile with the potential for this in mind and consider carefully what other personal information, such as photos, you post here. Remember to safeguard your professional image, which will be viewed by people you don't know and are likely to want to impress. The use of LinkedIn is now considered as essential to nurses who want career mobility as their resume, business card, and professional portfolio. See chapter 13 ("The Advertising Department of *You, Inc.*: Your Resume") for additional discussion of these tools.

Hobnopolis (www.hobnopolis.com)

Designed to be approachable for people 35 and older, Hobnopolis describes itself this way:

> An online community of professionals, people and just plain ol' townsfolk. The town is comprised of different areas of interest like jet-setting, golfing, music and so on. Each area contains immediate chat connections to others. Chat, interact, laugh, hobnob.
>
> The primary focus of the town of Hobnopolis is to break down barriers of communication for those people without a lot of time. Whether you're a jet-setting professional or a second-shifter, Hobnopolis will allow you to maintain a social life during your free time.

Listservs

Listservs are the predecessors of the social-networking sites described above. A listserv is a kind of electronic bulletin board comprised of special interest groups maintained by a university, association, or professional organization. On a listserv, you can post messages, ask questions, give answers, and track happenings. Listserv members communicate with each other via email and can choose only to read what everyone is saying or jump in with an opinion by posting a response to which someone else is likely to respond, creating a chain of communication about the topic.

There are thousands of listservs on many topics, such as music, sports, travel, dieting, politics, etc. To find a list of listservs, use any search engine, such as Google, and type in *listserv* plus your topic of interest. Take into consideration that some listservs are very active, resulting in a significant amount of email. Many nurses (perhaps you were one of them) tracked the September 11 attack by means of listservs. It became a way to participate without being there, to share in the experience, to receive and get support, and to hear from and rally behind New York nurses and those from other states who were directly involved in the efforts to help.

Email (Electronic Mail)

Email is the most familiar of the online networking tools. Email makes it possible for even those with the busiest of lives to establish and maintain personal and professional relationships, since staying in touch can be done from the comfort of your own home or another place of your choosing and at a time of your convenience. Portable technologies, such as telephones and personal digital assistants (PDAs), make sending and receiving email something you can fit into your other activities with ease.

Twitter

Launched in 2006, Twitter is an instant messaging system in which brief texts or web-based messages (called *tweets*) of up to 140 characters are sent to an identified list of followers. While its initial purpose was to keep friends and colleagues up-to-date about the tweeter's daily activities, it has become a widely used commercial and political tool to disseminate information and elicit feedback.

Nurses can use Twitter to stay on top of what is going on in the nursing community and to interact with each other and with other members of the healthcare team. Dena White, a health and well-being advocate who promotes nurses and the medical profession in the health sector, posted a blog titled "Top 10 Nurses to Follow on Twitter" (*health-image.com/health/top-10-nurses-to-follow-on-twitter/*). You can track the postings of these nurses and spread the word to your nurse colleagues through tweets of your own. Some of these nurses include the following:

Nursedotcom—Misty Turner is the director of Nurse.com. She also enjoys politics, social media, and networking.

Vickie_Milazzo—Vickie L. Milazzo of Houston, Texas, is known as the pioneer of legal nurse consulting, as well as being a best selling author. She has been training legal nurse consultants for more than 25 years.

Bob_the_nurse—A psychiatric nurse who is presently employed by a mental health drug team.

WorkingNurse—A great place to find job postings and interesting articles for nurses.

NurseAusmed—A practicing registered nurse from New Zealand who is also an avid blogger.

American Nurse Today, the official publication of the American Nurses Association, is one of many organizations reaching out to nurses. It offers Twitter updates on a wide variety of timely topics. You can subscribe by logging onto *www.twitter.com/amernurse2day*. Here are some examples of recent tweets:

- Nursing's role in healthcare reform. *www.americannursetoday.com/Article.aspx?id=7086&fid=6850*
- Nursing Peer Review within a Magnet facility. *www.americannursetoday.com/Article.aspx?id=7078&fid=6850*
- Detecting cardiac injury with telemetry. *www.americannursetoday.com/Article.aspx?id=7090&fid=6850*

PARTICIPATING IN NETWORKS

Many personal and professional needs can be met via networks, whether in person or online. Examples are provided in figure 12.2.

PROFESSIONAL NEED	TRADITIONAL NETWORKING EXAMPLE	ONLINE NETWORKING EXAMPLE
Track professional trends.	Attend your annual state nurses association convention.	Check the ANA website weekly *nursingworld.org*.
Find coaches and mentors.	Look around for possibilities within your current place of employment.	Join at least three nursing listservs; ask directly for coaches or develop relationships with nurses online that can lead to this kind of relationship.
Receive and give support, feedback, and encouragement.	Schedule regular meetings with colleagues to provide opportunities for this.	Schedule at least one "live chat" per week with nursing colleagues you work with or know from a listserv.
Earn continuing education credits.	Attend seminars and workshops on your days off and/or take advantage of what is offered in your place of employment.	Investigate the many online distance-learning sites with a wide range of topics.
Search for employment opportunities.	Call and/or tell everyone you know what kind of position you are looking for.	Explore the websites of organizations in which you are interested to determine if there are openings; post a message on a listserv asking for information and the experience of anyone who worked there.
Find the answer to a question about a procedure or technique about which you are unfamiliar and to which you are assigned the next day.	Call your nurse friends and colleagues; find your preceptor before you go home for the day.	Post a question on one of listservs; email your new nurse colleague in Alabama and ask him.

Figure 12.2

(*Contnued on next page*)

PROFESSIONAL NEED	TRADITIONAL NETWORKING EXAMPLE	ONLINE NETWORKING EXAMPLE
Participate in job fairs.	Schedule a day off and attend the job fairs you see advertised in the newspapers or in nursing publications.	Watch for virtual job fairs conducted online by employers (they are advertised in print publications and online); be prepared to submit your electronic resume and to be interviewed, or at least screened, as in traditional job fairs.
Submit your resume.	Hand resume out in person to colleagues or at a job fair.	Submit an electronic version of your resume online (see chapter 14 for how these differ from traditional ones).

Figure 12.2

NETWORKING TIPS

Create Time for Networking

Challenge your belief that there is no time in your busy life for networking, especially since you can participate in electronic networking anytime, anywhere. If you do not own a computer or have access to the Internet, make the purchase of this a professional priority or make use of public computers in libraries and schools. If you are still shunning technology and hoping to get by without it, keep in mind what was said earlier in the book: "In your nursing practice, while you may be able to choose low-tech versus high-tech work, there is no longer any such thing as 'no-tech.'" Feeling some degree of comfort with technology and use of the Internet is as relevant to your professional development as keeping your clinical skills and competencies current.

Give and Get

Networks are established to meet the needs of everyone in the network over a period of time. What you get and how much is sometimes determined by what you give. Pay attention to being a reciprocal partner in these relationships, and you will benefit enormously.

Be Proactive and Assertive

Take the initiative to establish conversations rather than always waiting to be approached. If this is not your strength, use networking opportunities to learn and develop it, practicing as you would any skill you were intent on learning. Consider seeking out a mentor or coach for assistance or reading a book about assertiveness. Or try talking with friends or coworkers who have conquered this fear and are now comfortable approaching others.

Present Yourself with Confidence

Create and rehearse a brief introduction of who you are, including a summary of your professional experience and/or personal interests. Consider talking about an achievement of yours that others would be interested in, especially if it is relevant to the topic of the networking event you are attending. In addition, take care about the image you are presenting to others as revealed in your manner of dress, your attitude, your speech and grammar, and so on. Be sure that what you post online reflects your professionalism and is respectful.

Formalize the Networking Experience

While networks can be formal or informal professional or social links, your approach to the process of networking should be formalized in that it is purposeful, organized, and focused on a purpose or goal you have set for yourself. The more structure you create around your networking experience, the more you will get out if it. Ways to formalize networking include the following:

- Conduct research to investigate which networks would best serve your needs.
- Participate in a variety of networks that represent your professional and personal interests.
- Bring along your business card (you do have one, don't you?) to exchange with others. It creates an impressive image and is also a way to keep track of whom you meet and whom you want to contact again. Chapter 13 contains information about business cards that you will find helpful. Establish a card file, traditional and/or electronic, to hold your contacts' cards that you can access when needed.

Increase Your Visibility

Attend meetings, join organizations, volunteer, and/or work on committees. Remember that networking is a mutual experience. Don't go to events just to see what may be in them for you. Determine what you would like to give as well.

Make Networks Work for You

When necessary, work at shaping the experience to meet your needs rather than complaining that the event you're attending or that networking in general doesn't work for you. If a proactive approach doesn't work, you may be in the wrong network; move on to others.

Practice Active Listening

Because networking is about mutuality, be a good listener, not just a talker. Try listening, as this anonymous quote reminds us, "because we have two ears and one mouth, we should listen twice as much as we speak!"

Consider Everyone You Meet a Contact

See the world anew, as a vast pool of networking possibilities, professional as well as personal. Then, smile, strike up a conversation, and look for opportunities to give and get information and support.

Smile, Smile, Smile!

It really does make a difference. You will look more approachable and, therefore, be approached more by others, which will make you feel good and result in making you smile even more! But you need to start this feedback loop by smiling.

Open Windows When Doors Close

Work on transforming rejection or defeat into potential opportunities whenever possible. For example, if a nurse recruiter closed the door on you, so to speak, by not hiring you for the position you wanted, try opening a window of opportunity instead. Keep in touch with the recruiter, perhaps by sending updated resumes periodically. Or consider striking up conversations with the recruiter at professional meetings you may be at together. In this way, the recruiter becomes a link in your network and a possible connection to other work opportunities.

Trust the Process

Make networking an adventure by trusting that the links and connections in them can eventually lead to opportunities that you may not be able to identify at first. Be optimistic by believing in a positive result. Keep the process going by attending meetings and nurturing relationships.

Online Privacy

Investigate how protected your online networking site is. Many sites erect safety measures (often called firewalls) to prevent nonmembers from accessing members' information. ANANurseSpace is an example of a protected site. Privacy concerns involve potential use of your profiles or postings by third parties for online and offline uses, such as advertising. Alternatively, consider the potential benefits of increased visibility for your professional development. As noted earlier, employment recruiters use networking sites as a tool.

Move Ahead with Caution

Recognize the potential pitfalls and professional implications when you use publicly accessed websites (such as Facebook) to discuss patient experiences and issues. Patient confidentiality is governed not only by the American Nurses Association Code of Ethics (*www.nursingworld.com*) but also by the Health Insurance Portability and Accountability Act (HIPAA). You can access a summary of the HIPAA laws at *www.hhs.gov/ocr/privacy/hipaa/understanding/summary/index.html.*

It is possible that HIPAA laws can be violated when discussing a patient, even when the patient not identified by name. Kathleen McCormac, RN, JD, a nurse attorney, addresses these issues in an article about the pitfalls and opportunities inherent in social media at Nurse.com (*news.nurse.com/apps/pbcs.dll/article?AID=2010108090045*). Ms. McCormac warns that because there isn't sufficient security on these sites, all material there can be used as evidence in legal matters. She advises nurses to find blogs and Listservs sanctioned by professional organizations (such as the American Nurses Association) to network and share ideas. Ms. McCormac also cautions against offering healthcare advice when using social media. She says, "You aren't covered by insurance when you do this; the person with whom you are communicating may live in a state where you are not licensed."

The bottom line when using social media is common sense, professionalism, and careful selection and use of your site.

CHAPTER 13

The Advertising Department of *You, Inc.*: Your Resume

WRITING YOUR RESUME

A resume advertises the nature of your nursing business, what your self-owned nursing practice, *You, Inc.*, has to offer. It creates the opportunities for dialogues with potential employers/purchasers of your nursing skills and competencies. A resume is an advertisement that may not directly get you a job but, like all advertisements, will call attention to what you have to sell. A well-written resume opens the door to the interview, really a sales process, which will be discussed in the following chapter.

A resume is a work in progress, the current representation of your professional nursing identity. Its style and content will grow and change over time, just as you and your work change. There is a reassuring autobiographical quality to a well-written resume that becomes a kind of mirror, reflecting where you have been and what you have done while it points the way to what you may do in the future. While employers may own your job and make decisions about its design and longevity, your resume represents what you own; namely, your work, your achievements, and your experiences. It represents what belongs to you after leaving the particular work environment in which those work experiences occurred.

To keep your resume up-to-date and ready for your next career move, review and update it approximately every six months, since futurists and forecasters say that significant changes affecting how you live and work are expected to occur with that frequency. This will give you a degree of reassuring control and preparedness during the state of permanent transition typical of today's healthcare workplace.

A resume is a summary of your experience and achievements worded in short phrases. It is not a job description. It is not a complete description of everything you've done. In fact, a well-written resume should create some questions—but not confusion—in the reader's mind, questions that could be asked of you in the interview. This gives you the opportunity to sell—to convince the employer that you have the nursing skills, competencies, and experiences needed. It allows you to emphasize the match between the employer and your abilities and, perhaps most importantly, to use the reactions of the interviewer to shape your responses.

Periodically revising your resume is a way to align and realign your professional identity, a way to remind yourself of where you've been and what your best experiences are. The process of writing a resume is likely to rescue from memory those skills and achievements previously overlooked. Revisions also give you the opportunity to rephrase and, therefore, realign your skills with current marketplace needs, thereby making you more employable. Many such realignments can be expected throughout your nursing career and, in fact, are a sign of a well-worn and potentially satisfying career path.

An excellent way to write or revise your resume is to create it with someone who can provide feedback and objectivity and help you shape it into the best possible sales tool. Consider working with a friend or colleague who has good writing skills and who can be objective about you. If you decide to use a professional resume writer or career coach, be sure you are involved in cocreating the resume. Allowing someone else to produce it in your absence denies you a level of involvement that serves to increase your confidence in *You, Inc.* and in the professional identity that your resume represents. If you choose to work on it alone, consider showing it to others for feedback.

Potential employers will be looking for a match between your credentials and experience on one hand and the requirements of the job they need to fill on the other. Choose your words carefully and economically. Too many words, repetitions, or irrelevant data will work against you and may even eliminate you from the pool of people being considered.

RESUME APPEARANCE

Your resume should be typed in a font typically used in business and professional documents, such as Times Roman or Arial. The size of the font should be 11 or 12 points. Avoid frilly, decorative fonts and use bolding, italics, and bullets sparingly.

Pay close attention to any special instructions requested by potential employers who may plan to scan your resume into a computer. Since the computer cannot accurately scan anything decorative, such as bullets or fancy fonts, ignoring these instructions may eliminate you from consideration. Generally, this is also true for resumes that are submitted online. More information about online resume submission will be provided later in this chapter.

The resume can be one to two pages in length but never more than two. Set the margins of the paper so that the information can fill the page with enough white space (empty space surrounding the typed words) to make for easy reading. Absence of white space indicates an attempt to cram too much material into too small a space, and for this reason, a two-page resume, when necessary, is advisable.

Use professional stationery with matching envelopes in white or off-white. It's acceptable to neatly handwrite the address on the envelope; in fact, a handwritten envelope may indicate a personal but still professional touch.

Keep in mind that there is no one way to write a resume. After following the generally accepted guidelines described here and elsewhere, the format is a matter of personal preference. The type of resume described here is called the reverse chronological resume, in which the most recent professional experience appears first. An alternative is the skill-based resume, or you might use some combination of both. Consult the Resources at the back of the book for more information about writing your resume. Select a style and layout you prefer and use it as a model for creating yours. Or model your resume after the style presented here.

GUIDELINES FOR RESUME PREPARATION

1. Contact Information

Place your name, credentials, address, and phone number centered on the top of the page. A line that separates this identifying information from the remainder of the text makes reading easier and quicker. Whether you choose to punctuate the initials of your credentials or omit the periods is a matter of personal preference; both are acceptable.

SALLY SMITH, BSN, RN
75 East Main Street #7A
New York, NY 10010
(100) 100-1000
Cell phone: (917) 100-0000
Email: sallynurse19156@aol.com

2. Profile or Summary of Qualifications

Use this in place of a job objective, which tends to limit how you might be seen. A job objective can be included in the cover letter that accompanies each resume you send out. Guidelines for writing a cover letter are included at the end of this section.

Waiting until your resume is completed to write the profile will give you a better sense of what you want to include. A profile is a summary, not a complete repetition of your resume. It should highlight your best features as well as the kind of characteristics that employers are looking for today.

Profile Examples

Here's an example of what a new graduate's profile might look like:

> Resourceful, recently graduated Registered Nurse with healthcare experience as a certified emergency medical technician ready to apply transferable skills, including triage and basic life support, to a lifelong interest in nursing. Excels in settings requiring independent decision making as well as team collaboration. Excellent organizational and critical thinking skills.

This is what a more experienced nurse might write:

> Highly motivated and resourceful Registered Nurse with demonstrated leadership and effectiveness in acute care hospitals and community-based settings. Possess solid and recent medical-surgical experience with a subspecialty in orthopedics. Excellent communication and critical thinking skills. Experienced in multidisciplinary committee work, including Magnet accreditation process. Capable of prioritizing multiple responsibilities in fast-paced environments.

3. Your Education and Credentials

If this section becomes too lengthy, consider including a portion of it after the description of your professional experience.

License and Certification

Identify the state(s) in which you are licensed. It is not necessary to include your license number. Instead, carry your license in your professional portfolio (to be described later in this chapter) and take it with you to the interview. Include professional board certifications from the American Nurses Credentialing Center (ANCC) and other professional associations.

Education

Place your education in reverse chronological order and include if you are currently enrolled. This section is for your formal nursing education, undergraduate and graduate.

Continuing Education

This is an extremely important selling and balancing feature to compensate for gaps or deficiencies in formal education or gaps in experience.

Professional Affiliations and Membership

This is another important selling feature, demonstrating professionalism, commitment, and leadership.

Special Abilities

Include foreign languages spoken, sign language, computer and Internet skills, and any other special talents.

Awards and Honors

This is no time for modesty. If you have these, say so. This might include membership in Sigma Theta Tau, the international honor society for nursing, or an outstanding nurse award.

Publications and Presentations

Mention any articles you may have written or any occasion where you were required to convey educational information to groups of people.

Here are examples of how these initial categories of your resume might look.

Examples of Education and Credentials	
License and Certification	Registered Professional Nurse, New York and New Jersey Certified Medical-Surgical Nurse, ANCC
Education	Bachelor of Science, Nursing, Adelphi University (in progress) AAS, Nursing, Salem Community College (2003)
Continuing Education	Basic Cardiac Life Support AACN Cardiology Education Update Case Management for Staff Nurses IV Certification
Professional Affiliations	American Association of Critical Care Nurses Sigma Theta Tau International Nursing Honor Society New York State Nurses Association
Special Abilities	Fluent in Spanish and American Sign Language Fluent in pen-based electronic documentation
Awards and Honors	Dean's List, Salem Community College (2000) Outstanding Academic Achievement Award, Salem Community College (2001) Listed in *Who's Who Among American College Students* (2002) Distinguished Nursing Practice Award, Circle Hospital Center (2003)
Publications and Presentations	Grand Rounds Presentations: Care of the Dying Patient, Brooklyn Hospital (2001) Nursing Grand Rounds: Mentoring of New Graduates, Brooklyn Hospital (2002). "Transition to Home Care for Acute Care Nurses" in *Advance for Nurses*, June 2001

4. Description of Your Experience

List your relevant jobs in reverse chronological order, with your most recent experience appearing first. Use one or more of the categories below to describe your experience:

- **Professional nursing experience:** Use this category to describe your work as an RN or nursing student.
- **Additional healthcare experience:** This is the category for jobs other than RN, such as LPN, nursing assistant, and emergency medical technician.
- **Additional work experience:** Mention work outside of healthcare here.
- **Volunteer work experience:** Use this category for unpaid experiences in areas of interest to you.

Guidelines for Describing Your Experience

When describing work experiences outside of healthcare, identify and then describe relevant transferable skills. Examples of transferable skills are triage of accident victims as an emergency medical technician or customer service skills as a bank teller.

Each description should include dates of employment, job title, and name and city/state of the organization (full address can appear on application, if necessary).

Start each description of your work experience with an action verb (see lists on pages 216 and 217) that begins a phrase that orients the reader to the size and nature of the agency for which you worked, as well as the general scope of your responsibilities.

Following this orienting phrase, write additional short and pithy phrases in "telegram style," rather than full sentences, that describe your most important responsibilities and achievements. Avoid repetition of experiences if similar responsibilities occurred in more than one job.

The list of action verbs that follows is divided into categories of job skills relevant to the descriptions you might be creating. Take a look at all the lists, as the verbs can often be applied to more than one skill set.

Communication Skills

clarified	communicated	conferred	defined
described	developed	explained	formulated
listened	lectured	referred	

Creative Skills

adapted	began	composed	conceptualized
created	designed	initiated	originated
performed	reshaped	revitalized	

Financial and Information Skills

accounted for	administered	appraised	assessed
budgeted	computed	forecasted	measured
planned	prepared	processed	projected

Helping Skills

advocated	assessed	assisted	cared for
coached	collaborated	contributed	diagnosed
educated	helped	provided	rehabilitated

Leadership Skills

achieved	assigned	completed	delegated
directed	expanded	headed	led
managed	pioneered	resolved	supervised

Management Skills

administered	coordinated	directed	established
improved	initiated	managed	organized
planned	produced	scheduled	supervised

Organizational Skills

charted	collected	distributed	executed
implemented	maintained	monitored	led
organized	prepared	provided	reviewed
scheduled			

People Skills

coordinated	collaborated	consulted	empowered
encouraged	facilitated	interacted	
motivated		participated	

Research Skills			
analyzed	collected	compared	conducted
critiqued	detected	determined	diagnosed
evaluated	formulated	gathered	identified
interviewed	investigated	located	organized
researched	searched		
Teaching Skills			
adapted	clarified	coached	developed
evaluated	facilitated	individualized	instructed
motivated	taught	trained	
Technical Skills			
adapted	applied	converted	designed
developed	maintained	remodeled	restored
replaced	solved	specialized	utilized

Examples of Professional Experience Descriptions

Example 1

Clinical Office Coordinator, Bronx Oncology Associates, Bronx, NY (7/01 to present)

- Provide nursing care and administrative support in a high-volume, 19 RN, 8 MD practice for the diagnosis and cutting-edge treatment of cancer.
- Perform telephone triage, including intervention and referral.
- Conduct independent nursing assessments and develop plans of care in collaboration with physicians.
- Provide education, counseling, and emotional support to patients and families.
- Act as liaison among patient, physicians, and healthcare institutions.
- Coordinate inpatient, outpatient, and office services, including the monitoring of plans of care to ensure compliance with insurance reimbursement policies.

Example 2:

Student Clinical Rotations, St. Joseph's School of Nursing, Staten Island, NY (6/09 to present)

- Learn and practice primary nursing care in collaboration with professional nursing staff and multidisciplinary team in a variety of clinical settings, including Med-Surg, ICU, CCU, ER, Pediatrics, Maternity, and Psychiatry.
- Develop, implement, and revise written nursing care plans, including discharge planning.
- Provide teaching and emotional support to patients and families.

Example 3:

Emergency Medical Technician, Brooklyn Emergency Medical Services, Brooklyn, NY (4/05 to 5/08)

- Provided prehospital emergency care for sick and injured patients as part of a two-person ambulance response team.
- Provided intervention at the scene, including triage, treatment, transport to treating facility, and status report to receiving staff.
- Initiated and maintained advanced cardiac life support, including defibrillation at scene and during transport.
- Acted as preceptor to newly hired emergency medical technicians.

Example 4:

Staff Nurse, Mount Olive Medical Center, New York, NY (3/00 to 9/02)

- Provided primary nursing care to adults with complex medical-surgical illnesses, often requiring critical care interventions, on a 40-bed unit specializing in oncology, pain management, and hematological disorders.
- Proficient in a broad range of critical care skills such as hemodynamic monitoring, ventilator care, titration of cardiac medications, and advanced life support.
- Responsible for written nursing care plans, including assessment and intervention of rapidly changing patient status.
- Assigned to frequent charge responsibilities.

Using the guidelines discussed, a completed resume might look like the example on the following page.

SALLY SMITH, BSN, RN
75 East Main Street #7A
New York, NY 10010
(100) 100-1000
Cell phone: (917) 100-0000
Email: sallynurse19156@aol.com

Highly motivated and resourceful Registered Nurse with current experience and a proven track record in providing nursing care for the stable and critically ill adult and geriatric patient. Capable of managing multiple assignments simultaneously and efficiently. Excels in environments requiring independent decision making and team collaboration. Able to interact effectively with management, staff, and patients from all levels and cultural backgrounds. Experience in hospital-wide committee membership.

License Registered Professional Nurse, New York State License

Education Bachelor of Science in Nursing, The City College of New York, NY (1986)

Continuing Education Basic CPR Certification; IV Certification; EKG and Cardiac Arrhythmias; HIV Nursing Care Strategies

Awards 1992 Nursing Employee of the Year, Oceanside Medical Center, New York, NY

Professional Memberships American Nurses Association, member
New York State Nurses Association, member

Additional Abilities Fluent in Spanish and American Sign Language
Computer competence includes Windows, pen-based documentation, and the Internet

Professional Experience

Staff Nurse, Radiology Department, Mount Olive Medical Center, New York, NY (7/94 to present)

- Provide primary nursing care during a broad range of radiologic procedures to in-patients and out-patients of all ages with medical-surgical problems.
- Manage the nursing care needs of stable as well as critically ill patients during and while awaiting procedures.

- Assist during complex procedures, such as MRIs and angiographies, including pre- and postprocedure assessment and support of patient well-being during procedure.
- Administer oral contrast material; insert and monitor IV during administration of IV contrast.
- Assess and manage allergic and life-threatening responses to procedures.
- Provide patient and family teaching, including emotional support.
- Participate in quality assurance activities, including patient surveys and documentation.

Staff Nurse, Intensive Care Unit, Oceanside Hospital, New York, NY (2/89 to 7/94)

- Provided primary nursing care to adult and geriatric high-risk patients with complex medical and surgical needs on a six-bed ICU with a ratio of one RN to two or three patients.
- Developed written nursing care plans, which included assessment and intervention of rapidly changing patient status, in collaboration with multidisciplinary team.
- Performed a broad range of critical care skills, including hemodynamic monitoring for patients with multisystem failure.
- Assigned frequently to charge responsibilities.

Staff Nurse, Medicine, Highview Hospital, New York, NY (2/86 to 1/89)

- Provided primary nursing care to adult and geriatric patients with medical and neurological problems on a 26-bed acute care unit.
- Responsibilities included nursing care plans, including discharge planning; patient and family education, including emotional support; multidisciplinary collaboration.
- Assigned frequently to charge responsibilities.

Online Resumes

Many employers scan your resume to store it in their databases. Depending on the scanning software, this process can dramatically change the readability of your resume. Older scanning software often doesn't recognize punctuation or decorative fonts or even some spacing features, such as centering. For this reason, when an employer specifies that you submit a scannable version of your resume or if you intend to submit your resume electronically (online), it is important to submit it as either a Microsoft Word document, an ASCII text file, or a portable document format (.pdf).

If your resume was created as an MS Word document, it is possible to convert it to an ASCII document by saving in that format rather than as a Word document (Use the "Save As" command). However, proofread the document once it is converted to be sure the content has not been altered in the conversion process. Sometimes words are run together and need to be separated to be clear.

COVER LETTERS

A cover letter needs to accompany the resume you provide to prospective employers. It is preferable to write a different cover letter for each employment situation, crafting it to target the qualifications you have that match that employer's needs. Once you customize one cover letter, it can be used as a template or model from which to create others. Yana Parker, in her book *The Resume Pro,*[1] suggests you think about the following questions to help prepare your letter:

- Why do you want to work for that organization?
- What do you know about the organization?
- How did you hear about it?
- What do you know about the position for which you are applying?
- How are you qualified for the position—what skills and competencies match the employer's needs?

Guidelines for a good cover letter, adapted from recommendations made by Parker, include the following:

- Address your letter to the person with the authority to hire you or who has been designated to interview you for the position (e.g., the nurse recruiter or other administrator). When unable to obtain this information, use a functional title, such as "Dear Nurse Recruiter," not "To whom it may concern" or "Dear Sir or Madam."
- Show that you know a little about the organization.
- Phrase your letter so that it is professional but still warm and friendly.

- Set yourself apart from the crowd. Try to find at least one thing about your skills, competencies, or experiences that is unique and relevant to the position.
- Be specific. State the position for which you are applying and how you heard about it.
- Be brief; a few short paragraphs, all on one page, will suffice.

An example of a cover letter follows on page 223.

IRIS CARTER, BSN, RN
35 Blossom Way
New Paltz, NY 10000
(100) 100-1000
Cell phone: (999) 900-0000
Email: ICRN19156@aol.com

January 17, 2011

Jill North, RN, MA
Director, Human Resources
New Paltz Hospital
7745 High Road
New Paltz, NY 12345

Dear Ms. North,

I would like to be considered for the position of psychiatric staff nurse in your acute admissions unit as you advertised in the *New York Times* on January 14, 2011.

I have a Bachelor of Science in Nursing with ANCC certification in adult psychiatric nursing at the generalist level. My most recent experience includes four years of psychiatric nursing experience in acute care as well as home care settings. Some of my accomplishments include

- participating in the opening of a new day care center for geriatric patients, including the orientation of newly hired nursing assistants;
- development of a standardized care plan for the confused patient; and
- serving on the nursing shortage task force.

Additional qualifications I can offer you are excellent communication and interpersonal skills and the ability to work independently and in team-based settings.

The enclosed resume describes my experience and credentials in greater detail, and I would welcome an opportunity to discuss it with you in person. I am available for an interview at your convenience.

I look forward to hearing from you.

Sincerely,
Iris Carter, BSN, RN

FOLLOW-UP LETTERS

A follow-up letter is an opportunity to reinforce a positive perception of you. It is a professional way to maintain contact. Because the interview is not unlike a sales experience, the more contact you have with the person contemplating your services, and the more positive a perception that person has of you, the more likely you will make the sale—meaning, land the job. Your follow-up letter should include the following components, adapted from Parker's *The Resume Pro:*

- An expression of appreciation to the interviewer for the opportunity to discuss and be considered for the job opportunity
- A reference to something that was discussed as a reminder and reinforcement of your experience, skills, and so on
- Additional information, or new reasons that you are interested in the job, perhaps based on what was discovered or exchanged in the interview
- An offer to provide additional information or participate in additional interviews conducted by others
- A clarification, when necessary, about something that was discussed in the interview, such as a question that was asked or an issue about which you want to add information
- An anticipation of hearing from the interviewer again, perhaps about a favorable outcome or at least about the decision that will be made

In the next chapter, The Sales Department of *You, Inc.:* Interview Skills, you will find a sample letter and more about interview follow-up.

BUSINESS CARDS

Business cards are a relatively easy and inexpensive networking and sales tool that make an impressive professional statement, potentially setting you apart from others. Carry them with you to exchange during seminars and networking events. End an interview with an assertive handshake, a warm smile, and a "leave-behind" in the form of a business card. Attach cards to copies of your resume to circulate at job fairs.

Sample Business Card

Iris Carter, BSN, RN
Registered Professional Nurse

35 Blossom Way
New Paltz, NY 10000

Telephone:	(100) 100-1000
Cell Phone:	(999) 900-0000
Email:	ICRN19156@aol.com

CREATE A PROFESSIONAL PORTFOLIO

A professional portfolio is a representative sample of your work, a collection of documents about who you are professionally and what you have to offer. It contains an accumulation of information related to your professional life—a historical chronology of your activities. It contains the documented elements and examples of your professional identity and experience, such as copies of your credentials, diplomas, and letters of reference and recommendation. Gathering them into one portable package organizes and safeguards them and allows you to carry them in a professional way to an interview.

Your portfolio can have a private and a public section. The private section can be used to safeguard and keep track of important professional documents, such as your license, certification information, and continuing education dates. You select from the private section of your portfolio what would be most relevant at a job interview. The public section is what you want others to see about you and what you have to offer. It's a sales tool, like a marketing book used by salespeople to demonstrate their wares. It may be tailored for the occasion by supplementing it with material from the private section of your portfolio, as indicated, and should contain the following:

- Broadcast letter that introduces you (similar to a cover letter but not targeted to one employer)
- Letters of reference and recommendation
- Typed list of three to six personal and professional references
- Your resume

- Business cards
- Copies of your professional credentials, including the following:
  - Diplomas
  - Transcripts
  - Continuing education certificates
  - Performance appraisals
- Samples of professional achievements and activities, such as these:
  - Letters of commendation or recognition
  - Articles you have published
  - Participation in poster sessions
  - Anything that documents your professional or personal accomplishments

Many nurses have long used a variation of this portfolio as a filing system to keep these professional documents both safe and accessible when needed. Today's business-savvy nurse takes this approach a step further and uses the portfolio as a sales tool, as a way to stand out from others. In addition, your portfolio becomes an important traveling companion to chronicle your career journey and keep the historical data about it organized. In some ways, it may serve as a way to reminisce and recount and then to feel proud about where you've been and what you've done. It can become the mobile equivalent of your own personnel file, similar to the one your employer keeps about you, serving to remind you of your accomplishments.

Your portfolio can be as creative and imaginative as you are and, in fact, is an actual demonstration to a potential employer of your creativity, confidence, and assertiveness. It can become a selling feature in and of itself! Consider using a colorful binder with interesting dividers. Take care, however, that it doesn't get too information-intensive, complex, or overdone; keep it professional.

Now that you have your advertising tools, set to go the next step is to use them as a sales tool. You will find this discussed in the next chapter.

CHAPTER 14

The Sales Department of *You, Inc.*: Interview Skills

The interview is your opportunity to present your best features to a potential employer, which translates into your credentials, experiences, skills, and talents. Your challenge is to convince this employer—to sell this employer—on the idea that you have what it needs. You want to convince the employer that it should buy what you have to offer, namely your ability not only to do the job but to excel at it, and that even though it may be considering other candidates, you're the one it should select.

TEST YOUR INTERVIEW KNOWLEDGE

Before reading further, determine your beliefs about interviews by placing a check mark in the box after each statement below to indicate if you think the statement is true or false. The answers, along with an explanation about each statement, appear at the end of this chapter.

1. ❐ True ❐ False To appear natural and spontaneous, it is better not to prepare responses ahead of time.

2. ❐ True ❐ False You should be cautious about your body language, because 40 to 50 percent of communication is nonverbal.

3. ❐ True ❐ False It is important to maintain direct eye contact at all times with the interviewer.

4. ❐ True ❐ False It is better to interrupt the interviewer than to forget to say or ask something.

5. ❒ True ❒ False Referring to a list when asking questions gives the impression of being unprepared.

6. ❒ True ❒ False Asking for a tour of the unit you may be working on appears intrusive.

7. ❒ True ❒ False Asking about the next steps or what your chances are of getting the job is too aggressive.

8. ❒ True ❒ False Writing a follow-up letter to the interview is redundant and a waste of the interviewer's time as well as yours.

9. ❒ True ❒ False If you decide to take another position before you hear the results of the interview, it's better to withdraw your application without saying why.

10. ❒ True ❒ False If you do not get the job, it is not a good idea to discuss the reasons why with the interviewer.

THE INTERVIEW AS A SALES EXPERIENCE

An interview is a sales experience in which the potential employer is your customer. In fact, the entire healthcare marketplace contains many potential customers to whom the nurse CEO of *You, Inc.* can consider selling the services of the self-owned nursing practice, namely nursing skills and competencies. Refer to chapter 8 for a discussion about how nurses are self-employed, even if they work for others.

Millie, a newly graduated nurse applying for her first job, provides an example of what selling can look like. She has just been interviewed for a position in the critical care unit of a major medical center that would provide her with a 16-week training and internship program. This organization accepts only eight candidates every six months, and Millie knows that more than eight people were interviewed. While she has been told that if she is not considered this time, she can reapply in the future, she doesn't want to wait that long. Recalling the interview, she remembered the nurse manager of the critical-care unit telling her that he expects 100 percent from his staff, so she wrote a follow-up letter saying, "You said that you expected 100 percent from your staff, and I want you to know that you can count on 120 percent from me." She included samples of two teaching tools she had developed as a volunteer for a health fair in which she had participated during her senior year, along with a description of her demanding student schedule, which included working part-time as a nursing assistant. Millie got the job. During the training program, the nurse manager told her how impressed he was by her persistence and motivation to pursue what she wanted. She had successfully sold him on the idea that she should not be passed over.

If the image of the pushy car salesperson or intrusive telemarketer interferes with your ability to "buy" the idea that you are selling during the interview process, consider a less stereotypical way to think about it so that you can benefit from this useful career strategy. Believe it or not, you already are a salesperson!

Selling is a natural part of all communication; in fact, sales pitches are inherent in almost all conversations. Every time you talk to someone about your point of view and every time you attempt to convince others to do something they may feel unsure of, an element of sales is involved. In fact, right now I am trying to sell you on the idea that selling is something that you can do, should do, and actually already do. I want you to buy this concept. And, right now, you may be acting like a salesperson, too, as you try to sell me on your point of view, perhaps that selling is incompatible with nursing practice.

If you still haven't bought the sales concept, or believe nurses don't/shouldn't sell, consider this. Teaching a new diabetic to give himself insulin injections when he is convinced that he will never be able to do so is a sales experience. Likewise, reassuring a new mother that she will indeed learn how to care for her first newborn is also selling. So is teaching sex education to adolescents and selling them on the need for protected sex.

The same element of persuasion that is involved in patient education or in much of your communication can be used on your own behalf in a job interview. Just as a salesperson can be a helpful ally when you are purchasing something you need but don't completely understand, so can you be helpful to your employer in your mutual quest for a satisfying and productive employment relationship.

WHAT SALESPEOPLE CAN TEACH US

If you take the best of what salespeople do and how they act, you have great guidelines for preparing and doing well in an interview. Typically, a salesperson doesn't expect you to buy what is being offered right away. The salesperson might first want to know more about you; perhaps send you free samples; create opportunities for you to become curious about what is being sold; and then answer your questions about it, ask you if keeping in touch would be okay, and so forth.

A good salesperson uses each of these contacts with the potential buyer to "close" the deal—to make the sale. In your case, closing the sale means landing the job. There are actually a series of closes before, during, and after the interview that move you closer to or further away from your goal of landing the job. Closes are like stages, and each one is a mini-success on the way to getting the job offer, which could be considered the final close.

The first close happens when you are offered the interview; it is the first yes to you from the employer and is based on the strength of your initial sales pitch in the form of your cover letter, resume, how you interact with the interviewer's assistant, etc. This means that about 50 percent of the interview process takes place before you walk in the door.

The interview is an appointment, sometimes brief, that is part of a much bigger process beginning with the very first contact you have with the potential employer. The interview is your opportunity to create a relationship with the buyer and not only sell what you have to offer but, as importantly, determine if you want to buy what the employer is selling in the job being offered. Thinking of the interview as a *reciprocal* sale empowers you to select the best nursing practice environment for your nursing product/service.

The second close might mean being offered additional interviews with other key members of the healthcare team with which you might be working, the nurse manager for example. The third close will be the job offer itself and whatever negotiations occur during that part of the hiring process that eventually lead both you and the employer to agree to the sale.

You may need to pursue each of these closes actively, as Millie did in the example that began this chapter. She did the work needed to sustain a potential employer's interest in her nursing skills and competencies by sending a letter following her interview, thereby continuing the dialogue and increasing her chances of making the sale; namely, getting into the critical care training and internship program.

Strategies for Success from the Sales Industry

- Accept that not everyone will be interested in your service or product.
- A percentage of people will buy it, perhaps 10 percent (one in ten).
- This percentage can change depending on the fluctuations in the marketplace that decrease or increase interest. For example, the nursing shortage has increased the percentage of people/healthcare organizations interested in purchasing the services of nurses.

- If one in ten of the people will buy, that means it may take nine nos to get to one yes. (This may be especially true in some areas of the healthcare marketplace. For example, there will likely be fewer nos in acute care than in ambulatory care.)
- On average, the more nos you get, the closer you are to the eventual yes, as long as you don't give up trying.
- Even if someone is interested, that doesn't mean that person will "buy" from you at that time.
- Because the potential to "buy" at a later date exists, staying in touch is essential to maintaining this future prospect and to building your professional network (as Millie did in the previous example).
- Objections to the purchase of your product/service may exist. Your challenge is to be ready for them, identify them when they occur, and then present information to overcome these objections. This does not mean overpowering or strong-arming the interviewer, as in the stereotype of the pushy salesperson, but rather convincing the buyer to think differently. An example for nurses might be highlighting transferable skills to substitute for skills or experience not yet achieved. How to anticipate these potential objections, some of which will come in the form of questions from the interviewer, will be discussed starting on page 233.

PREPARING FOR THE INTERVIEW

The interview is not a single event but a series of tasks and experiences that occur in three stages: preparing for the interview, the interview itself, and following up after the interview.

Learn about the Organization

The more you know about your potential employer, the better prepared you will be to do well in the interview, not only by responding well to the questions you will be asked but by appearing knowledgeable about the organization as well. Ways to familiarize yourself with the organization include conducting informational interviews (described next), exploring the employer's Internet website, seeking information through your personal or professional network, and determining if this employer has or is planning to seek Magnet status certification. Refer to chapters 2 and 3 for discussions about how organizations with this certification provide optimal practice environments for nurses.

Conduct Informational Interviews

An informational interview is not a casual chat with someone you just happen to meet but rather a planned experience in which you select one or more persons you hope will tell you about the position you are seeking, usually someone who is working in that organization or who has done the kind of work you want to be doing. It's a way to get the inside scoop.

The people you select to interview can be those you know or those who are referred to you by others (use your network here!). You can also find candidates for your interview online through a social networking site to which you may belong.

To get the most out of informational interviewing, tell the people you plan to interview in advance the purpose of the meeting and what you are interested in hearing about. This will give them the time they need to consider the most helpful responses for you. Prepare a list of questions, which might include the following:

- Do you enjoy your work? Are you doing what you expected or wanted to do when you considered this job?
- What does a typical workday look like?
- Describe the communication and relationships you have with your coworkers, with managers, with physicians.
- How are disputes and conflicts handled?
- What advice would you give to someone considering working here?
- Are you content with the choice you made? Have your expectations been met?

Add your questions here:

____

____

____

Determine If Your Qualifications Match the Employer's Needs

To prepare effectively for the interview, it is important to know how closely your nursing skills, competencies, and experiences match what the employer is expecting. Once you know this, you can compensate for what might be missing. If, for example, your IV and phlebotomy skills are five years old (experience is often not considered current after three years), taking a refresher course before the interview will go a long way toward reassuring the interviewer that you were aware of the need to update this skill and took care of it by being proactive, rather than thinking it might not be noticed or waiting to be told it would be necessary. Taking this action presents you as a responsible professional and communicates indirectly that you can be counted on to do the right thing, definitely an asset to any organization.

Refamiliarize Yourself with Your Resume

After you determine how closely you meet the requirements of the position you are seeking, review your resume to preselect what you want to highlight in the interview and to remind yourself what you might need to compensate for as well. This includes identifying your transferable skills and how you plan to weave them into the interview at an opportune time.

For example, let's say you are applying for a position as a direct care nurse in a psychiatric inpatient unit but have no formal experience as a psychiatric nurse. Your last position was on a medical unit in which you cared for a large volume of geriatric patients, many with dementia and depression. Let's further imagine that you not only enjoyed working with this kind of patient but, in addition, your peers and colleagues used you as a resource when these patients were assigned to them. Let's also add that you developed a standardized care plan for these patients that became the unit standard.

Using this scenario or one of your own, can you identify the transferable skills and competencies that could compensate for a lack of formal experience? List them here:

____

____

____

Anticipate Questions and Prepare Responses

The amount of time you spend considering questions the interviewer might ask and planning your responses will greatly influence the degree of comfort you have in the actual interview and, of course, how well you do. Remember, at least

50 percent of the interview process happens before you walk in the door, and a good part of that percentage is spent in this kind of preparation.

What follows are samples of questions you might be asked, along with examples of weak, ineffective responses to avoid and more effective responses that are could potentially sell you to the interviewer. It is unlikely that you will be asked all of these questions. Use them as a guide to prepare your own responses or as a kind of self-assessment that identifies your areas of strength or weakness. Use the interview preparation worksheet that starts on page 239 to develop your prepared responses to questions you believe you'll be asked.

Anticipated question: **Why do you want to work here?**
Ineffective response: You have good benefits.
Effective response: You have an excellent reputation for patient care, and I am ready for the challenges of an acute care medical center.

Anticipated question: **What makes you qualified to work on this kind of neurology unit?**

Ineffective response: I'm a hard worker.
Effective response: In my med-surg and community health rotations (in nursing school), I cared for many neurology patients. I liked the complexity of it, and my clinical evaluations from those rotations were excellent.

Anticipated question: **What are your strengths?**

Ineffective response: I like people, and people like me.
Effective response: I'm flexible and adapt quickly. I'm also a good organizer and work well with others.

Anticipated question: **What continuing education have you recently participated in?**

Ineffective response: A lot of different courses. Sometimes I send in those *AJN* tests, you know, those articles.

Effective response: I've just completed ACLS. I'm presently enrolled in IV certification. I'm planning to take an advanced physical assessment course in two months.

Anticipated question: **Tell me about your experience.**

Ineffective response: I've had experience in a lot of different areas, as you can see on my resume. (Note: Yes, the interviewer can read your resume. However, the interviewer also wants to hear you talk about it, so this is an opportunity for you to shine. A good resume should inspire questions in the interviewer's mind, giving you an opportunity to add to it, clarify, and shape your responses for the position you are currently seeking.)

Effective response: While I don't yet have RN experience, I have three years of hospital-related experience as a unit clerk and nursing assistant. My clinical rotations provided experience in all aspects of nursing, especially neurology patients, since we did our med-surg rotation on a neurology unit.

Anticipated question: **What do you want from this experience?**

Ineffective response: I want to work days, and I need health insurance.

Effective response: An opportunity to develop professionally, to share my ideas and skills. I am seeking new professional challenges. I also want to use this experience to qualify for ANCC board certification in med-surg nursing.

Anticipated question: **Why did you choose to become a nurse?**

Ineffective response: I like to help people.

Effective response: It's a profession that offers upward mobility, diverse challenges, and the kind of personal contact I've always enjoyed.

Anticipated question: **Tell me what you like to do best in nursing.**

Ineffective answer: Making people feel better.

Effective answer: I'm a good teacher, especially when it involves something complex like insulin administration. I know how to explain complicated things simply, and it's gratifying to experience people's response to it.

Anticipated question: **How do you deal with conflicts on the job?**

Ineffective answer: I never have conflicts. I get along with everyone.
Effective answer: I suggest that we discuss the issue to clarify the problem and check for misinterpretations. Conflicts are a natural part of the job, and good communication is essential to working them out.

Anticipated question: **If I were to call your former employer for a reference, what would she say about you?**

Ineffective answer: She would say I'm a good worker.
Effective answer: I believe she would tell you about my flexibility, especially when the hospital was downsized three years ago. There was a need for unit clerks to rotate to other units. While I did it to cooperate, I have to say that I gained a lot, too. It helped me improve my communication skills, since there was more contact with patients and family on the other units.

Anticipated question: **What do you think is most important about being a nurse?**

Ineffective answer: Never miss a day of work.
Effective answer: I believe nurses help people to heal themselves by supporting and sustaining them physically, mentally, emotionally, and spiritually until they can do this for themselves.

Anticipated question: **What are your work-related goals for the next five years?**

Ineffective answer: I'm not sure. I may be planning a family.
Effective answer: I would like to be ANCC certified in med-surg nursing and then begin thinking about graduate school.

Anticipated question: **Why should I hire you instead of other applicants?**

Ineffective answer: I have a lot of experience.
Effective answer: In addition to my familiarity with the hospital environment because of my work here as a unit clerk, I can offer you the same kind of commitment and flexibility that my last employer remarked about in my performance appraisal.

Anticipated question:	**Describe yourself.**
Ineffective answer:	I'm married, have two children, and work hard.
Effective answer:	I consider myself flexible and enthusiastic. I enjoy the fast-paced nature of acute care hospitals. I get along well with people of all backgrounds. I was recently inducted into Sigma Theta Tau (the international nursing honor society). I'm very proud of that.
Anticipated question:	**Why did you leave your former job?**
Ineffective answer:	I was bored.
Effective answer:	Overall, I liked my last job. However, I felt ready for the challenges of an acute care medical center like this one, especially because you specialize in oncology.
Anticipated question:	**Since you haven't worked in med-surg for some years, how well will you function here?**
Ineffective answer:	Once you've learned med-surg, you never forget it.
Effective answer:	I have kept up by taking online continuing education classes and recently completed a refresher course. I volunteer at a rehab center regularly. I've also kept up by reading *AJN* and going to professional conferences. In addition, I'm a fast learner and feel confident in my ability to do this job.
Anticipated question:	**Are you IV Certified?**
Ineffective answer:	No.
Effective answer:	No. However, I am currently pursuing certification and have experience in monitoring IVs and managing IV therapy.
Anticipated question:	**Have you ever managed a large clinic?**
Ineffective answer:	Not really.
Effective answer:	No, but I have successfully managed my brother's graphic design business. Some of my responsibilities were taking telephone orders and resolving customer problems and complaints. I also organized his telephone contacts and developed a filing system of his customers.

Anticipated question:	**Have you had experience in home visits?**
Ineffective answer:	Yes.
Effective answer:	Yes, during my nursing school clinical rotation. I enjoyed it. I liked the increased autonomy and the more comprehensive assessments that were possible in home environments.

Questions You Should Ask

It is likely that you will be given an opportunity to ask questions at some point during the interview, typically at the end. Should you think of questions as the interview is proceeding, inquire if you can ask them as they occur to you or if you should wait until the end.

It is always a good idea to ask questions. It demonstrates your professionalism and knowledge about important issues. Questions you could consider asking, especially if this information wasn't covered during the interview, follow. You might already know the answers to many of these questions, so it is not necessary or advisable to ask them all. Select the ones from this list that are most important to you.

- What is the role of the nurse in your organization? Or what are the expectations of the nurse in this position? To whom would I be reporting?
- For organizations without Magnet status: Is your hospital planning to apply for Magnet status?
- For organizations with Magnet status: Has Magnet status changed the role of the nurse in any way?
- Can you tell me something about the relationships the nurses in this organization have with peers and colleagues?
- Can you tell me about your staffing ratios and staffing policies?
- How has your organization been affected by the nursing shortage? Is your organization doing anything specific about it?
- Can you describe your inservice education programs, especially for new roles and responsibilities?
- What are the opportunities for and policies about advancement in your organization?
- Can you tell me about the salary and benefits? (Always make this the last question unless the interviewer brings it up earlier.)

Questionable Questions

The law prohibits the interviewer from asking you certain questions because they are discriminatory and not job related. These questionable questions include anything related to your

- age;
- marital status;
- children or childcare needs;
- nationality;
- ethnicity;
- sexual preference;
- religion; or
- financial status or credit issues.

INTERVIEW PREPARATION WORKSHEET

Step 1: Reflect on the job for which you are preparing to be interviewed and complete the following statements.

List the qualifications the employer is seeking.

____

____

____

Identify the qualifications you have.

____

____

____

Identify the qualifications you don't have.

____

____

____

Identify your transferable skills.

____

____

____

Step 2: After reviewing and refamiliarizing yourself with your resume and reflecting on your nursing skills and competencies, respond to the following questions.

Identify your strengths (What you excel at, love doing, have gotten great feedback about, have experience in, etc.).

____

____

____

Identify your weaknesses (What you are not good at, dislike doing, or have limited or no experience with, etc.).

____

____

____

Step 3: Identify how you plan to go about changing a weakness into a strength or how you will compensate for it.

____

____

____

Step 4: Develop a prepared response to describe one of your weaknesses.

____

____

____

Step 5: Develop a prepared response to describe one of your strengths.

____

____

____

Step 6: Develop prepared responses for additional questions you anticipate being asked.

____

____

____

THE INTERVIEW EXPERIENCE: TIPS AND STRATEGIES

It's natural to feel nervous about being interviewed. The strategies that follow will help you manage your anxiety and harness that energy for productive use on your own behalf.

Arrive Early

Be compulsive about this. Arrive at least one hour prior to the time of the interview to allow for unexpected travel delays or difficulty in finding the interview location once you have arrived. Upon arrival, go directly to the interview location so that you know exactly where it is and then find a place nearby where you can sit quietly until your appointment. Look for a coffee shop that is not too crowded or a nearby park or even a place of worship. You might also consider wandering around the block a few times if you are too restless to sit still.

Let Go and Rest/Relax

Utilize the same principle with which you might be familiar when preparing for exams: at some point, you need to let go, stop studying, and get some rest, trusting that all the preparation you have done will allow the needed information to emerge spontaneously at the right time.

Self-Care Prior to the Interview

- Get to bed early enough to feel rested on the day of the interview.
- Omit or decrease your intake of caffeinated beverages.
- Drink sufficient water to prevent dehydration from decreasing your energy or ability to think clearly.
- Breathe deeply enough, especially if you are anxious, to ensure your oxygenation is sufficient for thinking clearly.
- Eat breakfast, selecting foods known to give you high energy, usually some combination of protein and carbohydrates.
- Meditate, do a relaxation exercise, or just listen to relaxing music.
- Visualize, seeing yourself successfully asking and answering questions and then being offered the job.
- Use affirmations, saying something like "I do well in interviews," or "I can interview successfully," or "I am qualified for this job."

Carry a Briefcase

A briefcase or other professional carry-all enhances your image and keeps your documents organized. It should contain additional copies of your resume, your list of references and recommendations to give the interviewer, paper and pen, your list of prepared questions, a small bottle of water in case you need it, and your professional portfolio (see chapter 13 for a description of this important career tool).

Dress to Impress

Imagine the image you want to portray and then dress accordingly. You've heard it all before:

- First impressions are lasting impressions.
- A picture (your image) is worth a thousand words.
- Actions (and, in this case, appearance) speak louder than words.

Don't let your appearance detract from the quality of the work you did to prepare for this interview or from the qualifications you bring. Dress like the professional you are. Just because you may wear scrubs to work doesn't mean you should dress casually in the interview. Dress in a conservative manner. For women, this could mean a simple suit or dress with a conservative length, minimal jewelry, moderate makeup, stockings, low-heeled shoes, and a small handbag to accompany the briefcase in which you carry your professional portfolio. For men, this could mean a conservative suit and tie, white or neutral-colored shirt, polished shoes, and your portfolio. Both women and men should omit perfume or cologne or at least keep it minimal.

Display Confidence and Respect

When escorted into the office in which you will be interviewed, offer to shake hands (no limpness or shyness here!) and wait to be offered a seat. Greet the interviewer with minimal chatter and take your cues for responding from the interviewer.

Respond with Careful Thought

Keep your responses clear, direct, and succinct. Give enough information to answer the question but think carefully before offering what is not being asked. Find the balance between too much and too little.

Ending the Interview

Thank the interviewer for the opportunity of being considered for the position, offer to shake hands again, and (take a deep breath here!) ask what the next step is and what the chances of being hired are. This assertive, proactive question gives you the information you need for the important follow-up phase of the interview process. Asked appropriately, this question also portrays you as a confident professional. You may be pleasantly surprised by hearing of the intention to hire you (most likely following a check of your references) or at the very least what the next step in the process might be.

AFTER THE INTERVIEW

You're not done yet! There are two more very important steps to completing the interview process: the follow-up letter and an employer evaluation process in which you decide if this is the right position for you. Remember, the interview was a reciprocal process in which you *and* the interviewer got information. The employer might want you, but you may or may not want this employer.

The Follow-Up Letter

Writing a follow-up letter is a professional response to an important professional experience and is well worth your time and effort. To begin with, it gives you an opportunity to strengthen any weak responses you might have provided by replacing them with stronger ones after the interview when you are less anxious. This is demonstrated in the sample letter on page 246. The follow-up letter also reaffirms your interest in the position, if you are interested, or at least thanks the interviewer for the opportunity to be interviewed. This letter is likely to be kept on file along with your resume for a least one year and may benefit you in the future.

A Sample Follow-Up Letter

Iris Carter, a new BSN graduate, prepared for what she heard would be a very tough interview at an acute care hospital where she had her heart set on working. She knew (from the informational interviewing that she did) that she would be given a patient care scenario and asked to discuss how she would care for the patient. In the interview, the scenario she was given was the following:

> You are a nurse in the PACU (post-anesthesia care unit), and a patient who just had an abdominal hysterectomy is wheeled in from the OR. Give me two nursing diagnoses and two corresponding interventions for this patient.

Before proceeding, take this opportunity to imagine yourself responding to this question and write your answers here:

___

___

___

Iris's nursing diagnoses were related to the potential for bleeding and the potential for airway obstruction. After Iris offered several interventions for each diagnosis, she felt satisfied by her response. The interviewer appeared satisfied as well, since she went on with the interview.

When Iris reflected on the interview later, she realized she had forgotten one of the most important interventions of all, namely to check the patient's dressing for bleeding. Her initial panic subsided when she decided to include an explanation of this in her follow-up letter. At first, she considered ignoring the situation altogether, hoping the interviewer hadn't noticed or that it wouldn't matter. She rejected this idea as wishful thinking and rightly decided that ignoring it might do more harm than good. The letter Iris wrote follows.

Iris Carter RN, BSN
35 Blossom Way
New Paltz, NY 10001
(100) 100-1000
Cell: (917) 555-5000
Email: CarterIris12345@juno.com

Jill North, RN, MA
Human Resources Department
New Paltz Hospital
7745 High Road
New Paltz, NY 12345

January 12, 2011

Dear Ms. North,

Thank you for the opportunity to be interviewed for the position of direct care nurse in one of the surgical units of your organization. I learned a lot about what you expect from your staff and feel sure that I will meet your expectations. I especially liked the tour you provided. It allowed me to see the action I was hoping for and increased my desire to be part of a team like that.

In thinking back to the question you asked about the patient with the abdominal hysterectomy, I realized I neglected to tell you that one of my interventions would be to check the patient's dressing for bleeding. This is definitely something I would know to do, but I somehow omitted this step because I was a little anxious in the interview. I would welcome an opportunity to respond to any other questions you might have about my ability to care for this type of patient. As we discussed in the interview, my clinical rotations in nursing school included the care of many postoperative patients, and I have confidence in being able to care for them effectively.

I look forward to hearing from you.

Sincerely,

Iris Carter, RN, BSN

This letter says a lot about Iris's integrity and professionalism, as well as her sales ability. She portrays an image of someone who is concerned about quality patient care, as well as someone who is willing to take responsibility and to learn from her mistakes. It would be hard to imagine an interviewer not being impressed by this kind of response, whether or not Iris was offered the position.

EMPLOYER EVALUATION CHECKLIST

This final step in the interview process will help you determine if the position for which you interviewed is indeed what you want to accept, should it be offered to you. Use the checklist that follows to help you decide if a mutually satisfying match between you and this potential employer exists.

EMPLOYER EVALUATION CHECKLIST

Organization: ____

Date of Interview: ____

Contact Person: ____

Place a check in the box provided to indicate your satisfaction with the employment potential of this organization. The more checks that appear, the greater the match between you and the employer.

- ❐ The institution bases its policies and procedures on specified nursing standards.
- ❐ The institution has Magnet status certification or is in the process of obtaining it.
- ❐ You will be reporting to a nursing manager and/or nursing administrator (in general, this is preferred but not always necessary, as long as there is access to nursing resource people should the need arise).
- ❐ The roles and responsibilities of the position were clearly and adequately explained (check this statement twice if the description was given to you in writing).
- ❐ The nurse-patient ratio was described and is reasonable; there is an approved administrative mechanism to negotiate a potentially unreasonable assignment.

- ❐ There are opportunities for administrative and/or clinical advancement.
- ❐ The orientation for newly hired staff is adequate; there is a preceptor program.
- ❐ There is continuing education and on-site training, especially for new roles and responsibilities; education is encouraged; and some tuition reimbursement is provided.
- ❐ The starting salary for the position is satisfactory.
- ❐ The benefits package is satisfactory (health insurance, paid vacations, etc.).

Specify additional factors of importance to you on the following lines:

____

____

____

ANSWERS TO INTERVIEW QUIZ

The answers to the interview quiz earlier in this chapter appear below, accompanied by explanations. Use this information as a review of the material in this chapter.

1. False Preparation is essential for successful interviewing. It also helps you to lower your anxiety and manage your stress.

2. False A whopping 90 to 95 percent of communication is nonverbal and takes the form of body language; manner of dress; tone of voice; attitude; and behaviors such as punctuality, assertiveness, and so on.

3. False No one maintains eye contact 100 percent of the time. Looking away periodically and briefly as you ponder the answers to questions is normal.

4. False A better option is to jot down notes about questions you have and wait for the best opportunity to ask them, perhaps at the end of the interview or when asked if you have questions. However, use your judgment here. If you are confused, it's better to clarify this with a polite interruption rather than feel lost and unable to respond or continue.

5. False Just the opposite is true. Bringing a list makes you look prepared and interested enough to have given serious thought to this employment situation. It will also decrease your anxiety.

6. False This is an appropriate request. Taking a tour can provide a different and perhaps welcome source of data that words cannot completely convey.

7. False This is an assertive question that conveys confidence and professionalism. It is also an essential sales strategy for planning your follow-up and the focus of your efforts and energy. Assertiveness and productivity are essential characteristics, and it is well worth strengthening these skills.

8. False Not only does this kind of follow-up demonstrate that you know how to conduct yourself professionally, it also continues contact with the employer beyond the interview to keep your name familiar. In addition, it gives you the opportunity to strengthen weak responses caused by anxiety or insufficient preparation.

9. False A written letter expressing appreciation for the time and consideration granted you and a brief reason for your decision maintains the relationship and keeps the door open for future possibilities. It is a way to grow your network as well as your reputation.

10. False Asking this question could strengthen your approach for the next interview and may also keep the door open for the future should another position at that organization become available.

CHAPTER 15

The Most Essential Part of *You, Inc.*: The Resilient You

> "In a fast-paced, continually shifting environment, resilience to change is the single most important factor that distinguishes those who succeed from those who fail."
>
> —*Daryl R. Conner*
> *in* Managing at the Speed of Change*[1]*

The primary focus of this book so far has been strengthening the career management "leg" of your three-legged nursing career stool. Your professional credentials and experience comprise the second of these legs. This chapter focuses on the third leg, namely your personal needs, and asks the question: Are professional and personal needs mutually exclusive?

Your answer to this question can make all the difference in the achievement of a necessary work-life balance as well as having the energy, motivation, and resilience required for the ongoing evolution and development of all three legs throughout your career. While we might all agree that each of these legs needs to be equal to provide a strong enough foundation to support your nursing practice, translating this awareness into action can be tricky in a profession of mostly women and in which the needs of others are primary.[1]

ARE PROFESSIONAL AND PERSONAL NEEDS MUTUALLY EXCLUSIVE?

To start answering this question, let's consider the ideas of Gloria Steinem, who asserts that the needs of the individual are as essential as those of the group or the culture. In her book *Revolution from Within: A Book of Self-Esteem* (1992),[2] Steinem asserts that two revolutions are needed if the culture as well as the individual is to achieve egalitarian wholeness and equal opportunity.

The first revolution of which Steinem speaks is the well-known cultural movement she led in the 1960s against gender and racial barriers through the use of social and political action. Steinem later believed that a second, more personal revolution was just as important and equally essential to the success of the cultural revolution. She described this revolution as the enhancement of the *individual* spirit and consciousness required for self-development and sustaining one's core self-esteem.

She had initially believed that this kind of self-development was not required for cultural change to occur. In her book, she speaks of how she once scoffed at the human potential movement of that time, considering it unimportant to influencing the collective change for which she and others worked. Decades later, however, she became suspicious when she encountered women with too little self-esteem to take advantage of "hard won, if still incomplete opportunities and too many men who were addicted to authority and control as the only proof of their value." Both, she said, lacked faith in a unique self: that core self-esteem without which no amount of situational self-esteem can be enough. She eventually encouraged a dual focus: the individual *and* the collective. Both, she said, were essential; one without the other was incomplete and ineffective. For 21st-century nurses, Steinem's message translates into many dual commitments and simultaneous responsibilities:

- To yourself as an individual nurse as well as to the mission of healthcare employers for whom you work.
- To your own individual nursing practice and to the nursing profession as a whole.
- To your personal needs as well as the needs of the patients for whom you care.

To succeed in meeting these simultaneous needs means to experience the pull of polar opposites without resolving the dilemma in an either/or, black-or-white way. But it's certainly easier to choose one over the other—your needs or the patient's, for example. Many nurses have been doing just that for generations, reluctantly agreeing to overtime work, for example, when they know that they are well past their physical and mental capacities. Consider this question:

- What do you do to ensure that you have adequate nutrition, hydration, and rest periods when working a ten-hour shift, even if meal breaks are not usually taken by your peers because the workload is too great?

In the short run, giving up adequate nutrition, hydration, and rest periods seems like the easiest solution. In the long run, both optimal patient care and personal well-being would likely be jeopardized. While the needs of patients are clearly primary, ignoring your own needs on a regular basis will result in no one's needs being fully met and with patient care potentially compromised. The simplistic, short-term solutions of either/or, black or white, win or lose, and your needs or mine do not fully address the complex collision of needs that many nurses experience every day.

Because the culture of healthcare does not typically ensure that the needs of both patient and nurse are met, nurses who want both professional satisfaction and personal well-being must claim for themselves what they know is essential to quality patient care; namely, their own self-care. This may require engaging in your own personal revolution inspired by the hard-won experience and revelations of Gloria Steinem and others. Use the information in this chapter to take responsibility for this personal revolution or to strengthen the one in which you are already engaged.

WHAT MAKES NURSING PRACTICE STRESSFUL?

When nurses are surveyed about their work, they typically report feeling more stressed by their working conditions than by the patients they care for. Linda Aiken, the director of the University of Pennsylvania School of Nursing's Center for Health Outcomes and Policy Research, describes the degree of frustrated helplessness many nurses experience as related to persistent organizational problems heightened by the nursing shortage in which nurses are working longer hours with less help (Detroit Free Press, 2001).[3]

When nurses are unable to meet their responsibilities to their patients according to the standards of nursing practice to which they are held accountable, they experience a highly stressful conflict. Often, nurses respond to this conflict by developing patterns of behavior that tend to compound and amplify an already stressful situation.

For example, in an attempt to maintain safe and effective patient care in understaffed hospitals, they may work in a persistent state of stress with its heightened mental, emotional, and physical arousal during long shifts of 8 to 12 hours, often without taking adequate rest breaks to restore energy and frequently staying overtime to finish documentation and paperwork. Torn between the needs of their patients and their own needs, they often bypass common sense and choose the other person over themselves.

Consider the situation described below to determine how automatically you might respond to the needs of others, even if you know it's not the right action to take.

Imagine that you are on an airplane, traveling with a six-year-old boy who is clearly too young to care for himself and for whom you are therefore responsible. You've been in the air for about two hours and have settled down to a well-earned nap after a hectic morning of activity. You are awakened by lights flickering on and off and the plane jostling back and forth and realize you are flying through a thunderstorm. Suddenly the oxygen masks the flight attendants taught you how to use before takeoff drop down in front of you. Which of the responses below most closely matches what you would do?

1. I would put the child's mask on first because he can't do this for himself.
2. I would put my mask on first because unless I do, I may pass out, and then neither the child nor I would get oxygen.
3. I know I should put my mask on first, but my instinct is to put the child's on first, and it's hard to know if I could override this automatic behavior.

The correct answer, of course, is #2. However, many people find themselves more closely aligned with #3, knowing what they should do but torn about their ability to do it. Many nurses work without their symbolic "oxygen," which is of course, a metaphor for their physical, mental, emotional, spiritual, and interpersonal needs. They run around making sure everyone, their patients especially, have their "masks" on—get their needs met—but often neglect their own, even as they realize this behavior doesn't really make sense. This is an adapted behavior learned in response to conflict that is believed to not be resolvable with any other choice—the solution is others first and me last, if at all.

Managers and administrators who are squeezed tight by the economic restraint of managed care implicitly or explicitly reinforce these unhealthy, adapted behaviors by ignoring safe staffing ratios or implementing mandatory overtime polices. The exceptions are those healthcare employers with ANCC Magnet Accreditation (see chapter 2 for a discussion of Magnet Accreditation).

An additional factor that reinforces the behavior of overriding one's needs in favor of others is the fact that the nursing profession is comprised primarily of women (approximately 94 percent) who are culturally socialized to focus on the needs of others. Many of these women find themselves in the same relationship configuration in their personal lives, fulfilling the roles of wives, parents, and caregivers of their aging parents. Without developing the self-care skills required to ensure that their own needs are also met, these women are prime candidates for burnout and compassion fatigue.

RESPONSES TO STRESS

Stress is a highly personal experience. Whether or not a situation is experienced as stressful depends partly on the meaning this event has for you and on your lifetime of experiences, your perception and interpretation of the situation, and your unmet needs and expectations, among other factors. So while it may seem counterintuitive, the source of stress lies not fully in the event itself but rather in your unique interpretation of it. This is where you have more control than you may realize; you may not be able to prevent a stressful situation from occurring, but it is quite possible to manage your response to it and, as a result, feel less stressed even if the situation does not change. We will discuss one way to do this later in this chapter.

When stress is not self-managed, the potential for a crisis exists as the body-mind system exhausts its resources in response to the physiological and psychological arousal inherent in the stress experience. This is often compounded by escalating mental and emotional turmoil. As a result, you become flooded with external and internal stimuli. This diminishes your capacity to respond effectively.

The change inherent in all crises, whether of small or large magnitude, can be the result of happily anticipated events, such as the birth of a baby, or something unexpected, such as the loss of a job. Change can happen suddenly or unfold over a long time, slowly eroding your capacity to cope and forcing you to live with the kind of low-level stress known to contribute to burnout or compassion fatigue. An example of this could be the habitual foregoing of meal or rest breaks when working ten-hour shifts, leaving yourself without the fuel or energy for effective functioning. Change can escalate into a crisis.

The word *crisis* is taken from the Greek word *krinein*, which means turning point, a parting of the ways, a place of departure. Change and crisis have a lot in common, since both represent a departure from what was known towards something new and unfamiliar. In the Chinese language, the symbol for the word *crisis* is translated to mean the simultaneous occurrence of danger/threat and opportunity:

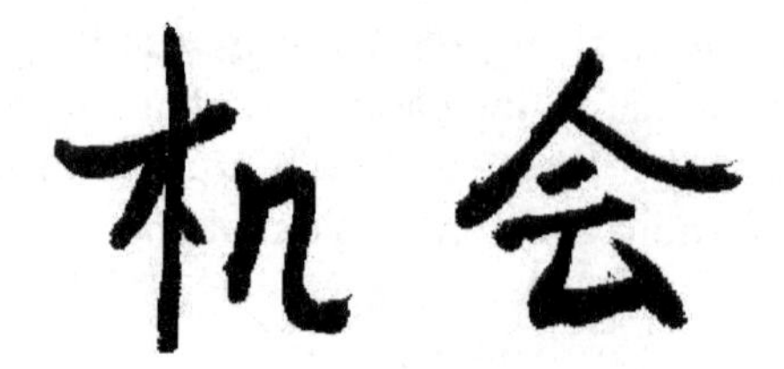

Crisis = Danger/Threat + Opportunity

There are three possible outcomes to a crisis or situation of change, all of which are greatly influenced by your ability to recognize the opportunity (rather than only the threat) that exists in it. Depending on the action you take, you could find yourself doing one of the following:

Thriving and growing as a result of it, perceiving the change as an opportunity, learning something new, increasing your personal and professional self-esteem

Surviving it, adapting without growing, going along with the flow, sticking it out, perhaps stagnating, not feeling fulfilled, looking for where the "grass may be greener"

Collapsing, feeling helpless, hopeless, giving up, regressing, believing you have been victimized, thinking you have been "done-to"

Three balancing features, shown in figure 15.1, are known to stabilize us in the midst of a crisis or change, influencing the degree of stress that will be experienced as well as the outcome that will result.

BALANCING FEATURES	QUESTIONS TO ASK YOURSELF
Accurate perception of the meaning and impact of the situation	Do you see the situation as a threat or a challenge?
Establishing and **using support systems** comprised of people and knowledge	Do you have or can you find people who can support you, to whom you can talk and feel heard? What is there to learn from this stressful situation?
Utilizing **coping skills** effectively to mediate the stress	Do you have routines, skills, and habits in place known to lower your stress, or are you willing to learn them? Examples include assertiveness, exercise, meditation, etc.

Figure 15.1

THRIVING ON CHANGE

Nurses are not immune to stress as a result of change. But the most successful among them will be thrivers, not just survivors. They know how to use change for their professional and personal growth. They navigate the difficulties and challenges that accompany change and come out winners. They often demonstrate leadership that brings others along with them.

How do you react in stressful or turbulent situations? Imagine yourself with a group of people in a boat rowing down a calm, peaceful river, when you unexpectedly find yourself in the rough turbulence of white water. The boat is tossed to and fro with dangerous half-hidden rocks and boulders around every bend. You didn't sign on for a white water rafting excursion, but here you find yourself nonetheless!

Permanent white water is a metaphor often used to describe the experience of navigating rapid, unexpected change. Three possible responses to this scenario follow. Which most closely resembles you or someone you know?

Responses to the White Water of Change

- **The Victim:** You expect the worst and believe that the danger you are sure is just around the next bend will do you in. You respond by being reactive rather than proactive. You spend a lot of time gripping the sides of the raft with white-knuckled terror, blaming and criticizing those trying to steer the boat. You fall into the water, requiring others to divide their attention between steering the boat to safety and rescuing you.
- **The Survivor:** You have your life jacket buttoned securely and know you will stay afloat if you fall into the water but believe you are only along for the ride. You think you have no choice about the direction of the boat or power to influence anything in the situation. Although you stay safely in the boat, you use all your energy holding on and contribute nothing to guiding the boat to safe waters.
- **The Navigator:** You see this unanticipated situation as a challenge. You are scared at times but get through the swelling currents by discovering skills you didn't know you had, developing new ones, or retooling old ones. Your confidence grows in proportion to your ability to work with those who are doing the steering. You save the Victim who falls into the water and reassure the Survivor whose anxiety is distracting those steering the boat.

It is not so much the intensity of a situation that determines whether you become a Navigator but the degree of control you believe you have over your predicament. Even Navigators sometimes find themselves pessimistic or wary and consider their glass to be half empty, so to speak. What makes them Navigators is their capacity to shift their state of mind from pessimistic to optimistic and then see the glass half filled. This capacity to shift perceptions and reinterpret the meaning of a situation distinguishes them from the Victim or the Survivor. It could be one of the best skills nurses could have in these complex times of constant change, uncertainty, and contradictory realities.

PROFILES OF NURSES RESPONDING TO STRESS

The following profiles describe the experiences of three newly hired direct care nurses who have just completed their orientation to the cardiac care center. They all find themselves faced with the same dilemma: they are working ten-hour shifts and discover that while meal breaks are assigned by the nurse manager, they are rarely taken by the staff, who cite the workload and patient acuity as too high to permit adequate break time. Which description most closely resembles how you might find yourself responding?

Profile of a Victim: Vicky

Although it is not her preference, Vicky feels obliged to do what others do and takes no meal breaks. She gulps glasses of water when she can and has learned to ignore the hunger pangs she feels toward the middle of her shift. She has developed headaches but does not connect them to her lowered blood glucose level or need for nutrition. She's also not sleeping as well as she used to.

She finds herself wondering why there is such a mental and physical frenzy among nurses in this unit, remembering that in the cardiac care center she just came from, meal breaks were routinely taken even though they had just as few nurses and just as many sick patients. She left that job because she felt harassed by a coworker who complained to the nurse manager that her change-of-shift reports were too long. She felt too intimidated to confront this coworker or seek assistance from the nurse manager. She had wondered about finding someone to talk to about the difficulties she was having but couldn't figure out how to go about it. She still wonders why her thoroughness was so misunderstood.

Seeing some of the same problems unfold at this new job, she begins to blame herself for leaving her last job, even though it felt like the right decision at the time. She feels preoccupied, sometimes depressed. She thinks she is powerless to react differently and doesn't see a way out of her situation. She is rarely aware that the needs and preferences of other people almost always take precedence over her own, and when she is aware, she doesn't know what to do about it. She finds herself discouraged and wonders if nursing was a good career choice after all.

Profile of a Survivor: Sam

Sam usually takes his meal breaks but spends them complaining and being angry because it is so difficult to do so. He is very critical of the nurse manager's organizational skills and leadership style and believes that the administrators of the medical center care more about their "bottom line" than the patients or the nurses who take care of them. He calls in sick frequently, telling some of his coworkers that he's entitled to these "mental health days" in exchange for the "abuse" he has to put up with working under conditions he believes are unfair.

He is assigned to be a preceptor for Tim, a new graduate, and seems unaware of the negative influence his attitude is having on him. He feels it is his moral responsibility to show Tim the "ropes" so he knows how to "play the game." He encourages Tim to think twice before responding to requests from peers for assistance if he wants to leave work on time. He declined to participate when the nurse manager asked him to attend a staff meeting to discuss how to develop a strategy for ensuring that nurses got their meal breaks, telling a coworker, "Why bother? Nothing ever changes around here. Anyway, that's her job, not mine." Sam waits impatiently for his next long weekend off or his vacation. He frequently talks about "putting in his time" until retirement.

Profile of a Navigator: Nancy

Nancy is new to cardiac care, having spent the first four years out of school on a general medical unit. While she found it very difficult to take meal breaks as a new graduate, she soon linked her afternoon crankiness and mental dullness to not eating lunch. At first, she tried having a snack while doing her morning documentation, but she soon realized that while she was sharper mentally as a result, she was still irritable. She eventually recognized that a short rest, along with nutrition and hydration, was essential for these long, intense workdays. Over a two-week period, she figured out how to organize her day around her patients' needs as well as her own. While her schedule is not ideal, even though she knows she is entitled to more, she now takes two or three 20-minute breaks on most days during her 10-hour shift.

She also decided to sign up for a relaxation class offered by the employee assistance program and now alternates visualization with meditation during her breaks. She also plans to use her iPod to listen to relaxing music during these breaks so that the noisy hustle and bustle of the unit is dampened.

During her three-month probationary evaluation with June, the nurse manager, the problem of meal breaks came up. Nancy was surprised to find that June felt as strongly as she did about the staff taking their meal breaks but was perplexed about how to continue encouraging them in the face of the resistance she met when she did so. June believed the reasons the staff gave her for ignoring their breaks were varied, including inability to organize their time, having trouble saying no, and problems delegating responsibilites. June believed that the staff indeed wanted meal breaks but couldn't figure out how to take them. As a result of the discussion with Nancy, June decided to have a staff meeting to discuss the issue and asked Nancy to share her personal struggles and solutions. Nancy agreed and also volunteered to post a notice about the meeting and to generate interest in it.

Nancy's initial feeling of achievement is being slowly eroded by the peer pressure she is experiencing from Sam, one of her coworkers, which started out as subtle criticism. Recently, he has become generally uncooperative and mysteriously unavailable to cover her patients during her breaks. Unsure how to handle this, she sought the advice of Mary, her preceptor for the first job she had after graduation and now her mentor. Mary helped Nancy realize that she would benefit from taking an assertiveness course and told her about one she had taken that helped her deal with the dysfunctional communication patterns that typify some groups of nurses. Nancy was fascinated by the term *horizontal interpersonal violence* used by Mary, who defined this as overt or covert hostility aimed at peers resulting from a sense of powerlessness in a situation coupled with not being heard by those in charge. She resolved to learn more about this destructive communication pattern after she completed the cardiac orientation next month.

The capacity Nancy has to navigate the challenges she faces will go a long way to ensuring a productive and satisfying career with the ability to lead others as well. Nancy's attitude, behavior, and self-awareness is characteristic of what is required of a successful nurse.

Burnout and Compassion Fatigue

Burnout is a form of mental, physical, emotional, and/or spiritual exhaustion that is not easily restored by sleep or rest. It is characterized by an inability to balance the demands placed on you with your capacity to meet them. Burnout results when stress management strategies fail. Nurses experience burnout as the result of feeling overwhelmed and unable to cope with the day-to-day stress of their work over a long period. These nurses are often wounded by the experience of caring too much about others while not knowing how to care enough for themselves simultaneously.

Compassion fatigue, which affects not only nurses but others in the helping professions, such as psychologists and social workers, is characterized by a loss of the ability to connect with or care about the emotional experiences of patients or other people in one's life. A kind of emotional numbness replaces the natural animation that once existed in response to the needs and experiences of others, resulting in avoidance of these situations or the robotic, going-through-the-motions behavior that is a compromise solution. Nurses continue in their work but are no longer able to experience or express the compassion they once felt. They join the ranks of the "walking wounded," continuing to work but feeling too stressed or too exhausted to care.

Valerie J. Nelson, in "Nurses and Burnout: What You Can Do to Prevent It" (*www.nurseweek.com/features/97-2/burn.html*), writes that Mickey Bumbaugh, MEd, a senior counseling specialist at M. D. Anderson Hospital in Texas

> thinks it's time to update the aging term [burnout], which was borrowed from the space industry. Instead of focusing on "avoiding burnout," she prefers to think of it as "learning to stay well."... The secret to having enough energy to keep giving compassionate care lies in creating a positive environment within yourself.... Don't forget to take care of yourself.[4]

Bumbaugh's advice to "create a positive environment within yourself" and "don't forget to take care of yourself" is a powerful antidote to burnout and compassion fatigue for nurses who use their skills as relationship builders in a cycle of caring that requires them mentally and emotionally to connect and disconnect, attach and detach to others—many, many others—in the course of a day, a week, and the years in a lifetime of work.

Nurses are particularly prone to compassion fatigue in understaffed healthcare settings, especially when there is insufficient recovery time from intense mental and emotional experiences. This dilemma leads to stressful conflicts or to the often-heartbreaking decision to leave nursing altogether. It is poignantly demonstrated in the following poem written by a nurse who chose to remain anonymous. The poem was a response to another well-known poem called "Crabbit Woman," which you can read at *pennyparker2.com/crabbit.html.*

Nurse's Response to Crabbit Old Woman

What do we see, you ask, what do we see?
Yes, we are thinking when looking at thee!
We may seem to be hard when we hurry and fuss,
But there's many of you, and too few of us.

We would like far more time to sit by you and talk,
To bathe you and feed you and help you to walk,
To hear of your lives and the things you have done;
Your childhood, your husband, your daughter, your son.
But time is against us, there's too much to do
Patients too many, and nurses too few.
We grieve when we see you so sad and alone,
With nobody near you, no friends of your own.
We feel all your pain, and know of your fear
That nobody cares now your end is so near.
But nurses are people with feelings as well,
And when we're together you'll often hear tell
Of the dearest old Gran in the very end bed,
And the lovely old Dad, and the things that he said,
We speak with compassion and love, and feel sad
When we think of your lives and the joy that you've had.

When the time has arrived for you to depart,
You leave us behind with an ache in our heart.
When you sleep the long sleep, no more worry or care,
There are other old people, and we must be there.
So please understand if we hurry and fuss—
There are many of you, and too few of us.

—Anonymous[5]

SELF-CARE FOR CHALLENGING TIMES

How, then, are we to succeed as nurses, indeed as people, in these challenging times of change, especially in circumstances that are less than ideal? Is it possible to sustain our strength, energy, and motivation while being bombarded with so much information, so many tasks, so many demands, and so much responsibility? How do we create the "positive environment within yourself" that Bumbaugh said is the "secret to having enough energy to giving compassionate care?"

What does it takes to succeed, to meet these challenges, to see the "turning points" in them, and perhaps use them as launch pads for our development and growth? Is this even possible?

It is not only possible, it is essential! Essential to each and every nurse, essential to the profession as a whole, and essential to the patients for whom the nurse cares. One way to meet these challenges is through the development of a self-care practice in which you learn to sustain your energy in complex situations, even if you can't influence the outcome of the situation in a way you might prefer at that time.

When a situation that causes stress cannot be readily changed, or when the solution is too far into the future to matter presently, what is still possible is to find a way to relate to the situation differently. It is still possible to find the meaning this situation has for you; to exploit some part of it on your own behalf; and to take charge of what you can, namely your responses to it, and use it for your benefit. What is quite possible is to take care of yourself through it, as Nancy did in the scenario presented earlier, and learn something about yourself as a result.

This does not imply agreement with the situation, nor does it rule out acting as a change agent when and where possible. Nurses have a responsibility to advocate for change and a proud history of doing so. Rather, what is being suggested here is an acknowledgment of what presently exists—of the reality in which you currently find yourself and at this moment cannot alter. This is not mutually exclusive with attempts to change the situation over time. It just means the time to change it may not be now. It is quite possible to disagree with what you are experiencing while not resisting the experience itself. Often, it is this resistance to an unpleasant reality that creates additional stress and tension. Try the experiment described below to play mentally with how this idea could work. You may be surprised at the results:

> Imagine you are walking down a busy street jammed with strolling tourists. Let's make it 42nd Street in New York City. Imagine further that you are in a great hurry to get errands done and no matter how fast you want to walk, you are blocked by groups of slow-walking, picture-taking, building-pointing tourists.

Most of you are likely to feel some tension arising in your body just thinking about this scenario. And it is this tension that is within our control. There is not likely to be a way to move these tourists along any faster, but there is a way to reduce your stress by practicing a kind of radical acceptance of the situation, which is different from accepting the behavior of these tourists.. You do this by taking a breath, surrendering to the reality you find yourself in, and slowing your pace. You "go with the flow," so to speak, and readjust your priorities.

Some of you might feel the tension in your body release a little just imagining this. You might want to try it and see what happens. It can work equally well when you're driving during rush-hour traffic. You are always free to take action at some point about this or any unpleasant situation if you desire. Or you might realize the futility of it and decide it isn't worth your time or effort. The point is to empower yourself to have that choice and, most importantly, to manage your experience of the situation.

This kind of self-focus, self-reliance, and self-care is essential not only to surviving but to thriving in challenging times. To decline responsibility for developing a self-care practice such as this is likely to contribute to burnout and compassion fatigue and to the diminishment of your motivation and passion for nursing.

SELF-CARE DEFINED

Self-care, like stress, is a very personal experience. What one person defines as self-care may be defined differently by someone else. Do you have a personal definition of self-care? Before reading the descriptions below, pause for a moment, consider yours, and write it here:

____

____

____

Self-care includes the capacity for self-awareness and self-management. Self-awareness is the ability to turn inward and hear the murmurs (or shouts) of discontent signaling the need for action on your own behalf. An example might be thirst or the need to decrease your sensory overload after a few hours of intense work. Self-management refers to the skills and strategies you employ to take this action (for example, reprioritizing your schedule or knowing how to respond to a coworker who always refuses your request to monitor your patients' IVs during your ten-minute break).

Self-care is

- the capacity to guide and regulate your mental, emotional, physical, spiritual, and interpersonal experience through difficult circumstances utilizing self-awareness and self-management.

- an ever-deepening practice that influences the process of growth and development, moving the mind, body, and spirit toward wholeness.
- stress management you can count on because it involves what you can control, namely your interpretation of and responses to people or situations.
- recognizing that it is not always necessary for situations or people to change for you to feel better.
- a key to work-life balance.
- an antidote to burnout.
- immunization against compassion fatigue.

EMPOWERMENT AND RESILIENCE

Empowerment is the refusal to be trapped without options—no matter what! Empowerment is you in the driver's seat of your life. Rather than following the advertising slogan of the Greyhound Bus Company—Leave the driving to us™—the empowered person responds to the call from Volkswagen—In life, there are passengers and drivers. Drivers wanted!™

Resilience is the capacity to bounce back from a situation that has the potential to overstretch or overextend your resources and capacities. It is the restoration of your mental elasticity, physical stamina, emotional buoyancy, spiritual strength, and interpersonal flexibility, all of which represent the holistic totality of your Self. The dictionary defines *resilience* as follows:

> Resilient, adj. (from the Latin, re = back + salire = to jump), 1. bouncing or springing back into shape, position, etc.; elastic. 2. recovering strength, spirits, good humor, etc. quickly; buoyant.

Think of the resilience of a rubber band that, when stretched, returns to its original shape and elasticity, able to continue its work of stretching again when necessary. Then think of a rubber band that is overstretched, perhaps for too long, and the loss of resilience that results. Have you ever had an overstretched rubber band break or snap on you? Consider this metaphor to determine how far you can stretch in a challenging situation and what self-care skills are required to recover your resilience.

Embracing a self-care philosophy fosters and includes the experience of empowerment and can result in the resilience and change-hardiness required of a successful nurse.

SELF-CARE STRATEGIES FOR BURNOUT PREVENTION

The self-care strategies that follow are loosely divided into holistic categories that overlap and are certainly not meant to be all-inclusive. Since self-care is always about tuning in to what is most important to you, use this list to whet your appetite to find more detail elsewhere. Use the resources at the back of this book to obtain more information. The self-care strategies below include the following categories:

- Major messages of self-care
- Physical self-care
- Interpersonal self-care
- Mental self-care
- Emotional self-care
- Spiritual self-care

Empowerment

The refusal to be trapped without options—NO MATTER WHAT!

Resilience

The restoration of your mental elasticity, physical stamina, emotional buoyancy, spiritual strength, and interpersonal flexibility by means of self-care.

MAJOR MESSAGES OF SELF-CARE

Never Abdicate Responsibility for Yourself

Take personal responsibility for maintaining and sustaining your own physical, mental, emotional, spiritual, and interpersonal energy. Expecting others to do so is a prescription for frustration, disappointment, and potential burnout. Your employer and others are always responsible for their actions, about which you are always free to disagree and of course to work towards changing if you desire. However, only you are responsible for your feelings and for managing your response to situations.

Make Your Self-Care Practice a Priority

Create space and time for it. Challenge beliefs that are inhibiting your ability to ensure that your needs are met, just as you ensure that the needs of others in your life are met.

Recognize That Your Self-Care Practice Is a Process, Not an Outcome

Self-care is not about perfection but about what you learn and how that changes you in the process. It is a continual, deepening discovery of who you are, what you desire, and how best to get it, if at all. Your self-care needs change as you grow and develop over time. Your appreciation of your own self-care and your periodic struggles with it can make you even more appreciative of the struggles others experience, including those of your patients. Model for them the process, the journey, of getting there rather than the potentially intimidating picture of perfect self-care. Perfection doesn't exist anywhere in the universe, including in your self-care practice.

Know Your Limits

There is a boundary between just enough and too much. This boundary is perhaps called "good enough." A boundary needs to be maintained between demands placed on you and your capacity to meet them. At a certain tipping point, quantity cancels out quality; the balance between both disappears and is replaced by a blurred flurry of mental and physical activity. Is it really true that "you can never have too much of a good thing"? If some chocolate cake is good, isn't it possible that too much of it can make you nauseous? If some spending gives you pleasure, can't too much spending land you in debt? And if some work is satisfying, can't too much lead to burnout?

Rise to the Challenge of Change

Expect change. Learn to adapt quickly to what's new and what's next. Learn to live with permanent transition by keeping your well-being self-generated rather than situation-dependent. An example of this is the self-employed attitude of the nurse CEO of *You, Inc.*, who knows that the employer only owns the job the nurse has temporarily consented to fill, not the very portable work the nurse does.

Perception Is Everything!

It can influence the intensity, duration, and outcome of stressful situations and their potential escalation into crises. How you think influences how you feel and eventually how you act, and your thoughts are something over which you have a great deal of control. Remember the pessimist and the optimist and their respective opinions about the glass being half empty or half full? It's not so much whether you feel optimistic or pessimistic, since both states of mind are natural to everyone at times. What matters more is remembering that you have the capacity to shift from one state of mind to another, from one way of feeling to another.

Treat Yourself with Love and Respect

Be patient and gentle, loving and generous, with yourself as you guide yourself through your self-care practices. It's not easy to unlearn patterns of behavior that might be keeping you from doing what you know is in your best interest (for example, learning to say no to additional responsibilities).

PHYSICAL SELF-CARE

Get Your "Oxygen"

Remember the story about the oxygen mask on the airplane earlier in this chapter? Find ways to get your symbolic "oxygen" just as you go about your day making sure everyone else gets theirs. This might include nutrition, hydration, and deep breathing as you race down those hallways. Or it might mean learning to say no to additional responsibilities that overstretch your resources.

Breathe, Breathe, and Breathe!

Check in with yourself periodically throughout your busy workday. How are you breathing? Busy people under a lot of pressure tend to take shallow breaths because muscle tension keeps their chest from expanding fully. You know the effects of shallow breathing on the amount of circulating oxygen required for precise thinking and mental alertness. You would be very concerned if one of your patient's oxygenation was compromised. You would take immediate action. In fact, you would treat this as an urgent situation, perhaps even an emergency. Remember to translate this knowledge to yourself as well.

Movement and Exercise

Include exercising and movement as a part of your self-care practice. No one needs to remind you of all the health benefits that exercise provides or what an essential stress management strategy it is. There is no way to do the rigorous work nursing requires without maintaining your physical stamina. Do whatever you have to do to get motivated to establish an exercise routine that works for you.

Eat Well

Adequate nutrition is essential for your body and mind to function well. It's needed for mental clarity and for protection against fatigue. You know this. You learned it in nursing school. You teach it to your patients. Be sure you apply this to yourself as well. Don't fool yourself into thinking you can calculate medication doses or multitask all that technology accurately without it!

You could try simple diaphragmatic breathing by allowing your breath to flow in and out of your abdomen, imagining it as a balloon, or you could try slowly counting your breaths or even a walking breath mediation. See "Take a Break, Catch a Breath" written by Colleen Wenrich, RN, (*www.nurse.com*) for an excellent discussion on how to do this as well as how to incorporate it into your work day.

Sleep and Rest

Make sure you get enough sleep and rest or, if you can, nap regularly. Sleep is not a disposable commodity, even though many of us act as if it is. Think for a moment: What's often the first thing you do when pressed for time to get an overdue project done? If your answer is to get up earlier or stay up later, consider the effect this has on you and try organizing your time differently or, at least, scheduling time to compensate for lost sleep at some point.

Manage Your Time

Take time management seriously. Recognize that it is just as important to prioritize your schedule as it is to schedule your priorities. To make sure that self-care practices are one of the priorities, schedule them into your day and week. Get a planner or a calendar and use it to ensure that self-care has a place, as well as other appointments and errands. You are much more likely to get to the gym, shop for nutritious foods, or keep your "play dates" if they are scheduled into your life rather than placed on a mental to-do list that is easily forgotten.

INTERPERSONAL SELF-CARE

Detach and Unplug

Detach from others periodically. Slow the pace once in a while. Dare to spend a day in your pajamas every so often! Challenge yourself to unplug from all the technology you are tethered to and overstimulated by day in and day out.

Imagine that not knowing what is going on in the world for 10 or 12 hours might be more restful than checking on the Dow Jones average from your Palm Pilot or tracking that ubiquitous "crawl" along the bottom of your TV screen. Using the voice mail option on your cell phone could allow you to manage technology rather than allowing it to manage you.

Seek Solitude

Find a sanctuary for you alone, at home and at work, and use it. Even if it's only for five or ten minutes, use it! Find a space you can go to, however briefly, to recenter and reground yourself and breathe more fully. Look around your workplace. What about the grounds surrounding the hospital? How about going outside briefly and combining solitude with a little stroll or a fast walk? There are lobbies and bathrooms everywhere. Be creative. This isn't about locking yourself away from your responsibilities for hours on end. This is about taking a few moments and quieting yourself down, treating yourself to a few minutes of solitude, to feel restored so you can do more. If this still sounds impossible, read the next self-care practice.

Say Yes to Yourself

Learning to say no to others more often allows you to increase the times you can say yes to yourself. Establishing realistic boundaries ensures that you have your needs met at least as often as you meet the needs of others, including your patients, your coworkers, and the nurse manager who is desperate and counting on you to stay overtime just one more day this week. If this feels impossible, take an assertiveness course or consider psychotherapy to sort out why you have difficulty treating yourself with the same consideration and respect you are willing to give to others.

If you still find it impossible to imagine taking your meal breaks, and nothing you've read in this book or elsewhere has convinced you, consider this additional way to think about it. Most organizations do not pay employees for the 60 to 90 minutes that are allotted for meal breaks. For example, if you work from 8:00 AM to 4:30 PM, you are most likely getting paid for seven or seven and a half of these hours. When you don't take the allotted time for your breaks, you might as well compute your hourly rate and drop off that amount of money in an administrator's office as a donation to your employer. If you do this every day you work, you are making a substantial donation to this organization. If you are getting overtime pay for working through your meal breaks, consider the effect this has on your physical and mental well-being.

Don't Play the "Blame Game"

Hold other people responsible only for their behavior, not for the feelings you have as a result of that behavior. Anger doesn't fully happen as a direct cause of someone doing something that you didn't like. It's much more complicated than that. A major source of anger is in the meaning the situation has for you.

Blaming someone for how you feel is not just taking the easy way out, it's also an abdication of the responsibility you have for yourself. There's a lot of power in the feeling of anger, especially when used on your own behalf. Knowing what you want (a key to why you may be angry in the first place) and then harnessing the power in it to use on your own behalf is empowering and growth enhancing. For a wonderful discussion of realigning your understanding of anger in this way, read *The Dance of Anger* by Harriet Lerner, especially the chapter titled "Who's Responsible for What, the Trickiest Anger Question of All" (see Resources).

Manage Conflicts, Don't Run from Them

Recognize the value in conflict that occurs naturally in healthy relationships. When managed well, conflict serves to strengthen relationships rather than weaken them. Conflict occurs when there are opposing points of view. Hearing about the views of others allows you to modify your own view and to grow and learn as a result.

Whenever many people are together trying to do something complicated (deliver good patient care, for example), conflict can naturally arise. When it is welcomed in the spirit of hearing opposing views, situations are eventually shaped in a better way than one person's ideas alone could ever accomplish. Explore conflict management strategies that allow you to contribute your ideas as well as hear the ideas of others.

MENTAL SELF-CARE

Imitate Willow Trees

If you don't like something, change it. Be proactive. Be assertive. Rally the troops around you. Take charge. Show leadership. And, after all is said and done, if you can't change it, change the way you think about it. Adapt to what is there, not what you wish could be. It's okay to keep working on what you want to be different, as long as you also accept what is in front of you. As discussed earlier, this doesn't mean giving up in defeat and accepting a compromised situation but rather making a shorter-term decision to "go with the flow," to imitate flexible willow trees instead of rigid oaks, as you continue your efforts toward the longer-term process of change.

Monitor Your Inner Dialogue

Work towards creating a positive attitude within yourself. Monitor your self-talk, your inner dialogue, that chattering you hear in your head that accompanies you through your activities. How you think about what you are doing will definitely affect how you feel. For example, as you are trying to learn a complicated procedure, replace "This is so hard; I'll never learn it," with "I know I'll get this if I just stay focused and keep trying. I've learned other complicated procedures. I can learn this one, too." Yelling at yourself creates stress and tension and prevents you from learning. You wouldn't yell at patients who were struggling to learn how to give themselves insulin. Neither should you yell at yourself, even if no one but you can hear it.

Use the Power of Affirmations

Consider using affirmations to create a positive and encouraging inner environment. An affirmation is a statement, a series of words, stated in the present tense, that you repeat silently to yourself again and again. The power in an affirmation comes from the repetition of it, which eventually influences what you believe and becomes self-fulfilling. Every nurse has the potential to be great, to excel, to contribute, and to have a satisfying and fulfilling career. What contributes enormously to these outcomes is your belief in yourself. Try the affirmations below and use the Resources section at the back of the book to learn more.

- "I am proactive and assertive."
- "I can prioritize and organize my time well."
- "I am able to provide for my self-care needs at work."

EMOTIONAL SELF-CARE

Allow Your Feelings to Strengthen You

Make space for and allow feelings to have a prominent and private place in your life. You are exposed to and a participant in some of the most powerful human experiences and personal dramas to be found anywhere. It is a myth that nurses get used to the pain and suffering they witness. To get used to it means to detach from it, and that only happens when burnout prevents you from being able to be caring and compassionate because it just hurts too much.

Pain, yours as well as others', is part of the fullness of life. Feelings unexpressed do not go away. They get transformed into other experiences, such as muscle tension, headaches, explosive reactions, overeating, loss of mental clarity, and so on. This is not to suggest that you let your feelings have free rein anytime, anyplace. It is often important to shift from them and focus on the task at hand, something nurses are quite good at. What they are often less good at is shifting back again to those feelings at another time and allowing the release that accompanies the expression of feelings to reduce the harmful effect unexpressed feelings can have.

SPIRITUAL SELF-CARE

Experience the Beauty and Peace of Meditation

Meditation is so much more than getting quiet and focusing on your breath. It is a quiet state in which the body's metabolic rate slows. It is different from sleep and can actually be more restful in some ways. Meditation is both a stress management strategy and a personal development tool. There are so many ways to meditate, including walking meditations, that it would be impossible not to be able to find one to suit you.

The beauty of meditation is that when you turn inward and get quiet, you can be with yourself in ways that are impossible as you go through your sensory-overloaded and "other-focused" day. Turning inward allows you to determine how to guide yourself according to what's right for you rather than for others. Take a course or find someone who meditates and allow that person to share how precious an experience meditation can be.

Try Prayer

If it fits into your spiritual and religious beliefs, try making prayer a part of your life in a regular way. Many people experience a kind of restful meditative state when praying. Spirituality is about being in the presence of the spirit that is a part of you and experiencing its beauty and immense power. Yoga is considered by many to be a spiritual experience, a way to access the spirit through the body. Nursing practice has a spiritual component to it that is separate from the religion of the patient for whom you are caring. You learned this in nursing school. Clearly, it is true for you as well.

CREATE SPACE IN YOUR LIFE FOR SELF-CARE

This chapter has provided you with a road map to the territory of self-care practices that you can explore in more depth at your own pace. Create your own itinerary, lingering longer at some destinations, moving on or returning to explore more fully at other times, following whatever path takes you to your current and evolving interests and needs.

The question that began this chapter was: Are professional and personal needs mutually exclusive? You are invited to answer that question for yourself, to reflect seriously on it and allow responses to emerge over time as you ponder this idea and experiment with self-care practices designed to address the complexity of your experiences. Become aware of how your answers evolve in keeping with the deepening of your professional and personal growth.

Do whatever is required to take your self-care practice as seriously as you take your other-care skills. Use the resources in this book and others you may already have around you. Find role models and mentors. Those who journey down this road will go a long way to ensuring that they have the resilience and personal power required for a long and satisfying nursing career. To remind you to say *yes* to yourself more often and to make space for your self-care in your life, consider the following poem.

The Art of Disappearing

When they say Don't I know you?
say no.

When they invite you to the party
remember what parties are like
before answering.
Someone telling you in a loud voice
they once wrote a poem.
Greasy sausage balls on a paper plate.
then reply.

If they say We should get together
say why?

It's not that you don't love them anymore.
You're trying to remember something
too important to forget.
Trees. The monastery bell at twilight.
Tell them you have a new project.
It will never be finished.

When someone recognizes you in a grocery store
nod briefly and become a cabbage.
When someone you haven't seen in ten years
appears at the door,
don't start singing him all your new songs.
You'll never catch up.

Walk around like a leaf.
Know you could tumble any second
Then decide what to do with your time.
—Naomi Shihab Nye[6]

Appendix

ENDNOTES

Chapter 1

1. Dickens, Charles, *A Tale of Two Cities.* Saddleback Educational Publishing, Inc.
2. US Census Bureau "Health Insurance Coverage 2006." *www.census.gov/hhes/www/hlthins/hlthin06/hlth06asc.html.*
3. Kirschheimer, Barbara, "Wrestling with a New Reality." *Nursing Spectrum,* 7/14/08
4. Joaquin Barnoya and Stanton Glantz. "Modifiable Behavioral Factors as Causes of Death." *JAMA* 2004; 291: 2942–2942.
5. Ellis, Rhema, Interview of 2002 Graduates. *The News with Brian Williams,* June 7, 2002.
6. "Nurses for a Healthier Tomorrow." Campaign News. *www.nursesource.org/campaign_news.html*
7. *Report: The Official Newsletter of NYSNA* (35) 2, 2005.
8. Cataldo, Jackie, "Smoke and Debris." *Journal of the New York State Nurses Association,* Spring/Summer 2002, Volume 33, Number 1, p. 25.
9. Stevens, Janet, "Someone to Fill My Shoes." *Nursing Spectrum,* June 3, 2002.
10. Naisbitt, John, *Megatrends: Ten New Directions Transforming our Lives.* Warner Books, 1982.

Chapter 2

1. Gordon, S., *Life Support: Three Nurses on the Front Lines.* New York: Little, Brown and Company, 1997.
2. Nightingale, F., *Notes on Nursing: What It Is and What It Is Not.* London: Harrison and Sons, London, 1859. (A facsimile edition: Philadelphia: J.B. Lippincott Company, 1946.)

3. Henderson, V., *Basic Principles of Nursing Care*. London: International Council of Nurses, 1961.
4. American Nurses Association, *Nursing's Social Policy Statement—The Essence of the Profession (2010 Edition)*. Silver Spring, MD: Nursesbooks.org, 2010.
5. —— *Nursing's Social Policy Statement* (2010 Edition). Washington, DC: Nursesbooks.org, 2010.
6. —— *Code of Ethics for Nurses with Interpretative Statements*. Washington, DC: American Nurses Publishing, 2001.
7. —— *Nursing: Scope and Standards of Practice*. Silver Spring, MD: Nursesbooks.org, 2010.
8. New York State Nurses Association, *Nurses' Rights: Preserving Nursing Practice in Unsafe Client Patient Situations*. Latham, NY: NYSNA, 1997.
9. American Nurses Association, *Enhancing Quality of Care Through Understanding Nurses' Responsibilities*. Kansas City, MO: ANA,1986.
10. Fagin, C. Claire M. Fagin Papers, Center for the Study of the History of Nursing, School of Nursing, University of Pennsylvania. Available from *www.nursing.upenn.edu/history/collections/fagin.htm*. (Accessed on May 16, 2008).
11. New York State Nurses Association, *Nurses' Rights: Preserving Nursing Practice in Unsafe Client Patient Situations*. Latham, NY: NYSNA, 1997.
12. *Memo for CMA Executive Directors on Nursing's Agenda for the Future*. Washington, DC: ANA, 2002.
13. Buerhaus, P., Auerbach, D.I., and Staiger, D.O., The Recent Surge in Nurse Employment: Causes and Implication. *Health Affair*, 2009; 28: 657–668.
14. U.S. Labor Department, Bureau of Labor Statistics. *Registered Nurses*. Available from *www.bls.gov/oco/ocos083.htm*. (Accessed on May 16, 2008)
15. Murray, M., "The Nursing Shortage: Past, Present and Future." *JONA 32*, (2002).
16. Kimball, B. and O'Neil, E., *Health Care's Human Crisis: The American Nursing Shortage*. Princeton, NJ: The Robert Wood Johnson Foundation, 2002.
17. New York State Nurses Association. *Assessing Your Nursing Practice Environment: A Guide for Nurses Seeking Employment in Health Care Settings*. Latham, NY: NYSNA, 1997.
18. McClure, M., Poulin, M., Sovie, M., and Wandell, M., *Magnet Hospitals*. Kansas City, MO: American Nurses Association, 1983.

19. Sigma Theta Tau, *Honor Society Study Shows Majority of Nurses Rely on Evidence-Based Practice*. Available from *www.nursingsociety.org/Media/Pages/EPBrel.aspx* (Accessed on May 20, 2008).
20. Committee on Quality of Health Care in America, Institute of Medicine, *Crossing the Quality Chasm: A New Health System for the 21st Century*. Washington, DC: National Academy Press, 2001.
21. Melynk, B., and Fineout-Overholt, E., *Evidence-Based Practice in Nursing and Healthcare—A Guide to Best Practice*. New York, NY: Lippincott Williams & Wilkins, 2005.
22. Aiken, L. et al.. Hospital Nurse Staffing and Patient Morality, Nurse Burnout, and Job Dissatisfaction, *JAMA*, 2002; 20.
23. Needleman, J. et al., Nurse-Staffing Levels and the Quality of Care in Hospitals, *New England Journal of Medicine*, 2002; 346.
24. American Association of Critical Care Nurses. *AACN Delegation Handbook* (2nd ed.) Washington, DC: AACN, 2004.
25. American Nurses Association. *ANA's Health System Reform Agenda*. Silver Spring, MD: Nursesbooks.org, 2008.

Chapter 3

1. Conner, Daryl R., *Managing at the Speed of Change: How Resilient Managers Succeed and Prosper Where Others Fail*. New York: Random House, 1992.
2. "Faculty Shortages Intensify Nation's Nursing Deficit." American Association of Colleges of Nursing Publications. *www.aacn.nche.edu/Publications/issues/IB499WB.htm*
3. "A Continuing Challenge: The Shortage of Educationally Prepared Nursing Faculty." American Association of Colleges of Nursing Publications. *nursingworld.org/ojni/topic14/tpc14_3.htm*
4. "Nursing Education's Agenda for the 21st Century." American Association of Colleges of Nursing Publications. *www.aacn.nche.edu/Publications/positions/nrsgedag.htm*
5. Joel, Lucille, "Education for Entry Into Nursing Practice: Revisited for the 21st Century." *nursingworld.org/ojin/topic18/tpc18_4.htm*

Chapter 4

1. Thede, Linda Q Informatics and Nursing: Opportunities and Challenges, 2nd ed. Lippincott, Williams, Wilkins, 2003, p. xi and p. 200

Chapter 5

1. Benner, Patricia, *From Novice to Expert: Excellence and Power in Clinical Nursing Practice.* New Jersey: Prentice Hall, 2001.
2. Leddy, Susan and J. Mae Pepper, *Conceptual Bases of Professional Nursing.* New York: JB Lippincott Company, 1993.
3. Kramer, Marlene and Claudia Schmalenberg. *Path to Biculturalism.* Nursing Resources, 1993, p. ix.
4. Narrowing the Gap in Nursing Shortage Due to Influx of Older First-Time Nurses January 13, 2007 *www.medicalnewstoday.com/printerfriendlynews.php?newsid=60608.*
5. Testimony of the Americans for Nursing Shortage Relief (ANSR) Alliance to the Subcommittee on Labor, Health and Human Services, US House of Representatives, March 31, 2006.
6. Engels, Nicholas, "One Solution to the Nursing Shortage: Second-career Trainees." *The Business Journal of Milwaukee,* April 23, 2001. *milwaukee.bizjournals.com/milwaukee/stories/2001/04/23/focus2.html*
7. Quinn, Rose, "Second Sight." *Advance For Nurses*, July 22, 2002. *advancefornurses.com*
8. Wood, Debra Anscombe. *A Guide to Mentorship by and for Managers. www.nurse.com* 2/25/2008.

Chapter 6

1. Deutsch, Claudia. "A Longer Goodbye" in the *New York Times* Special Section on Retirement, April 21, 2008, p. 1.
2. "Workplace of the Future: Spotlight on the Mature Nurse Workforce." Proceedings Report, June 22, 2005. Wieck, K. Lynn, "Retaining the Older Worker/Mature Nurse Survey Findings 2003–2004. *www.leadsummit2007.org/cemter/pubs.htm.*
3. Center for American Nurses. Mature Nurse & Nurse Retention Resources pdf, 2008, page 2. *www.centerforamericannurses.com*
4. Bureau of Labor Statistics Occupational Outlook Handbook: Registered Nurses, 2008–09 edition. www.bls.gov/oco/ocos083.htm.
5. Buerhaus, PI, Steiger, DO & Auerbach, DI (2000) "Policy Responses to an Aging Registered Nurse Workforce." *Nursing Economic$,* 18(6) 278–303.
6. Berlin, LE & Seachrist, KR. "The Shortage of Doctorally Prepared Nursing Faculty: A Dire Situation." *Nursing Outlook,* 50(2) 50–56.

7. Yordy, Karl, The Nursing Faculty Shortage: A Crisis for Health Care. *The Robert Woods Johnson Foundation, Spring 2006.*
8. Frauenheim, Ed, "Grey Matters." *Nurse Week*, January 22, 2001, page 4–5. *www.nurseweek.com/news/features/01-01/mature.asp.*
9. Domrose, Cathryn, "Bridges Across Time." *Nurse Week*, May 14, 2001. *www.nurseweek.com/news/features/01-01/mature.asp.*
10. Freedman, Marc. *Encore: Finding Work That Matters in the Second Half of Life*. Perseus Book Groups, 2007, page 91. and page 118.
11. Bonifazi, Wendy L. "5 Minutes with Ardis Martin, RN, MSN." *Nursing Spectrum,* November 5, 2007.
12. Gibran, Kahlil. *The Prophet.* 91st edition, Alfred A. Knopf, 1973, p. 27–31.
13. CNW Group: Fidelity Investments. "Attention Business Editors: If You Work in Retirement, Are You Still Retired?" *www.newswire.ca/en/releases/archive/December2006/11c5502.html?view=print. page 1.*
14. Dychtwald, Ken as quoted in "Retire on Less Than You Think," revised edition by Fred Brock, Times Books, 2004, p. 10.
15. Phillips, Kelly. "Hospitals Must Make Accommodations to Retain, Recruit Older RN's." *www.nursezone.com/print/Articles.aspx?ID=12579&profile=Spotlight+on+nurses. Page 1*
16. Sherman, Rose O. "Leading a Multigenerational Nursing Workforce: Issues, Challenges and Strategies. *The Online Journal of Issues in Nursing (OJIN),* page 1 and 2. *www.nursingworld.com.*
17. Childers, Linda. "Welcome Back: New Programs Encourage Retired and Former Nurses to Return to the Workforce." September 20, 2004, *www.nurseweek.com.*
18. Frost, Robert. *Mountain Interval.* New York: Henry Holt & Co., 1920; Bartleby.com, 1999, *www.bartleby.com/119/.*

Chapter 7

1. Health Resources and Service Administration. (March 2010) Initial Findings from the 2008 National Sample Survey of Registered Nurses. Retrieved June 22, 2010, from *bhpr.hrsa.gov/healthworkforce/rnsurvey/initialfindings2008.pdf*
2. Wilson, Bruce, "Men in American Nursing History." *www.geocities.com/~brucewilson/*
3. National Advisory Council on Nurse Education and Practice. (2001). First Report to the Secretary of Health and Human Services and the Congress. Retrieved on May 26, 2008 from *bhpr.hrsa.gov/nursing/NACNEP/reports/first/5.htm*

4. Guteri, Gail O. (2008). "Men & Women in Nursing." *Advance for Nurses* (April 28, 2008). Retrieved May 2, 2008 from *nursing.advanceweb.com/Editorial/Content/PrintFriendly.aspx?CC=113152*
5. American Association of Colleges of Nursing. (2001). "Effective Strategies for Increasing Diversity in Nursing Programs." *Issues Bulletin,* December 2001. *www.aacn.nche.edu/Publications/issues/dec01.htm*
6. Williams, Michael, "President's Notes: A Journey of Rediscovery: So How Does It Feel to You?" *AACN News*, August 2001. *www.aacn.org/AACN/aacnnews.nsf/GetArticle/ArticleThree188?OpenDocument*
7. O'Lynn, Chad E. (2007). Gender-based barriers for male students in nursing education programs. In Chad E. O'Lynn & Russell E. Tranbarger (Eds.), *Men in nursing: History, challenges, and opportunities* (pp. 169–187). New York: Springer.
8. Williams, Ashleigh and Nikki Battle, "Breakthrough to Nursing." *NSNA Imprint*, Feb./Mar. 2002.
9. Williams, Debra, "Looking For a Few Good Men." *Minority Nurse*, Spring 2002.
10. Evans, Michael, "The Image of Nursing: Past, Present and Future." *NSNA Imprint*, Feb/Mar 2002.
11. Sigma Theta Tau International Honor Society of Nursing. (1997). "Woodhull Study on Nursing and the Media." *www.nursingsociety.org/Media/Pages/woodhall.aspx*
12. Bernard Hodes Group. (January 26, 2005). "Men in Nursing Study." New York: Hodes Research. Retrieved May 27, 2008 from *www.hodes.com/industries/healthcare/pdfs/MenInNursing2005.pdf*
13. Culp, Mildred L. (2008). "Stereotypes down for male nurses." *New York Daily News* (May 13, 2008). Retrieved May 15, 2008 from *www.nydailynews.com/money/2008/05/12/2008-05-12_stereotypes_down_for_male_nurses.html*
14. Snel, Alan, "Paradise Lost No More." *Advance For Nurses*, June 24, 2002
15. Bennet Swingle, Anne, "Still Not Much of a Guy Thing." *Hopkins Nurse* (a publication of the Johns Hopkins Hospital), Fall 2001.
16. "Nurses for a Healthier Tomorrow." Campaign News. *www.nursesource.org/campaign_news.html*
17. Nursing Management/Bernard Hodes Group, *Aging Nurse Workforce Survey*. New York: Bernard Hodes Group, 2006.
18. The Campaign for Nursing's Future." Johnson & Johnson. *www.discovernursing.com*
19. Ekstrom, David N. (2008). "American Assembly for Men in Nursing." In H. Feldman (ed.), *Nursing leadership: A concise encyclopedia* (pp. 34–35). New York: Springer.

20. The American Assembly for Nursing (AAMN). (2008). AAMN Foundation Scholarships. Retrieved May 26, 2008 from *aamn.org/scholarships.html*
21. Williams, Debra. (2006). Recruiting men into nursing school. *Minority Nurse* (Winter 2006). Retrieved May 23, 2008 from *www.minoritynurse.com/features/men/03-21-06e.html*
22. Leighty, John. (2007). It's a guy thing: The number of men in nursing school is on the rise. *Future Nurse* (Fall 2007), pp. 14–16.
23. O'Lynn, Chad. (2008). *Monterey Peninsula College receives grant to retain nursing students. Interaction* (Official Publication of the AAMN), *26*(1), 1, 7.
24. Rosenstein, Alan H. (2002) "Nurse-Physician Relationships: Impact on Nurse Satisfaction and Retention." *American Journal of Nursing, 102*(6), pp. 26–34. Retrieved May 26, 2008 from *nursingcenter.com/library/JournalArticle.asp?Article_ID=278949*
25. Mason, Diana. (2002). "MD-RN: A Tired Old Dance." Editorial, American Journal of Nursing, 102(6), p. 7.
26. Whitman, Walt, "The Wound Dresser." Selections From "Leaves of Grass." New York: Avenel Books (Crown Publishers, Inc.), 1961.

Chapter 8

1. Bridges, William, *Job Shift: How to Prosper in a Workplace Without Jobs*, New York: Addison-Wesley Publishing, 1994.
2. Saltzman, Amy, "You, Inc." *US News and World Report,* October 28, 1996. *arguscoaching.com/usnews19961028*
3. Noer, David, *Healing the Wounds: Overcoming the Trauma of Layoffs and Revitalizing Downsized Organizations.* San Francisco: Jossey-Bass Publishers, 1993.

Chapter 9

1. Jones, Laurie Beth, *The Path: Creating Your Mission Statement for Work and Life.* New York: Hyperion, 1996, p. 3.
2. Covey, Stephen R., *The 7 Habits of Highly Effective People.* New York Simon and Schuster, 1990, p. 106–107.
3. Cabrera, James C & Charles F Albrecht Jr. *The Lifetime Career Manager: New Strategies for a New Era,* Adams Media Corporation 1997.

4. Perkins-Reed, Marcia, *Thriving in Transition: Effective Living in Times of Change*. New York: Touchstone: Simon and Schuster, 1996, p 173.
5. Fritz, Robert. *The Path of Least Resistance.* Fawcett Book Group, 1989.

Chapter 10

1. Bureau of Labor Statistics, *Occupational Outlook Handbook: Registered Nurses,* 2010–11 edition. *www.bls.gov/oco/ocos083.htm*.
2. DeBack, Vivian, "The New Practice Environment" in *Nurse Case Management in the 21st Century*, New York: Mosby, 1996.

Chapter 11

1. Benner, Patricia, From *Novice to Expert: Excellence and Power in Clinical Nursing Practice*. New Jersey: Prentice Hall, 2001.

Chapter 13

1. Parker, Yana, *The Resume Pro*. Ten Speed Press, 1993.

Chapter 15

1. Conner, Daryl R., *Managing at the Speed of Change: How Resilient Managers Succeed and Prosper Where Others Fail.* New York: Random House, 1992.
2. Steinem, Gloria. *Revolution From Within: A Book of Self-Esteem.* Little & Brown Co. 1992.
3. Bergstrom, Bill, "Almost Half of Nurses Near Burnout, Study Shows." *Detroit Free Press,* May 7, 2001. *freep.com/news/health/nurse7_20010507.htm*
4. Nelson, Valerie, "Nurses and Burnout: What You Can Do to Prevent It." *Nurse Week. www.nurseweek.com/features/97-2/burn.html*
5. Author Unknown, "Nurse's Response to Crabbit Old Woman." Penny's Place in Cyberspace. *pennyparker2.com/crabbit.htm*
6. Shihab Nye, Naomi, "The Art of Disappearing." *Words Under the Words,* 1995.

RESOURCES

INTERNET RESOURCES

Internet resources are included throughout the book as references or as suggestions for learning more. For example, chapter 4 is packed with useful websites for clinical, professional, and technical reference.

Because Web addresses tend to change and listings on the Internet are frequently added or deleted, knowing how to use search engines to find a topic of interest is useful and important. Below you will find a list of general interest and nursing-specific search engines along with Internet gateways and portals that will provide you with annotated, searchable databases including hyperlinks directing you to your sites of interest.

General search engines include *www.google.com*, *www.yahoo.com*, *www.altavista.com*, and *www.excite.com*, to name a few. Enter keywords representing your topic of interest into any of these search engines, and they will access databases and documents available online and provide you with lists of links to them.

Nursing-Specific Internet Gateways, Portals and Search Engines

www.nurse.com
The publisher of *Nursing Spectrum* and *Nurse Week*, advertising periodicals free to nurses, provides search engines along with job listings, professional news, dates of career fairs and continuing education (CE) events, CE self-study courses, and social networking sites, including blogs and listservs.

www.nursingworld.org
The official website of the American Nurses Association provides updates and information on all areas of professional nursing practice, including health policy, political activism, print and online publications, and more, as well as opportunities for social networking and links to all state nurses associations.

www.nursingcenter.com
This is a portal to more than 800 continuing education activities and clinical articles for 50 leading nursing journals published by Lippincott, Williams and Wilkins, including the *American Journal of Nursing, Nursing 2008, Nursing Management,* and many specialty journals.

www.nursing-portal.com
This is a nursing search engine for sites around the world with a database of 20,000 nursing links.

wethenurses.com
Provides global online information to the nursing community, including links to job opportunities, nursing schools, publications, and news.

PRINT RESOURCES

Nursing: Historical and Contemporary Writings

Florence Nightingale Today: Healing, Leadership, Global Action. Barbara Montgomery Dossey, Louise C. Selanders, Deva-Maria Beck, American Nurses Publishing, 2005. Dossey extends and advances our knowledge of Nightingale as the founder of modern nursing into the 21st century by illuminating how her ideas, theories, and work provide the foundation for health science, health statistics, social reform, and evidence-based practice as well as holistic nursing, nursing theory, and public health.

Florence Nightingale: Mystic, Visionary, Healer. Barbara Montgomery Dossey, RN, MS, HNC, FAAN, Lippincott, Williams & Wilkins, 2000. A unique and beautifully illustrated biography of the founder of modern nursing who was a trailblazing social activist, decades ahead of her time.

Nursing, The Finest Art: An Illustrated History. M. Patricia Donahue, PhD, RN, The CV Mosby Company, 1996. A beautifully illustrated history of nursing from ancient to modern times set in its social, political and economic contexts. Documents the alternating presence and absence of men in nursing.

Life Support: Three Nurses on the Front Line. Suzanne Gordon, Back Bay Books, 1998. Suzanne Gordon, who is not a nurse but an award-winning journalist, is aptly described as a champion and advocate of nurses, believing that nurses are at the foundation of the healthcare industry but often invisible and without enough of a voice. In this book she relates how she followed nurses at Beth Israel Hospital in Boston for three months. She says of this experience that "what she learned is that rather than being a lesser form of doctoring, nursing is a highly developed profession with care-giving skills completely separate from those of doctoring but it is undervalued because nurses are generally women" (*Lubbock-Avalanche Journal,* 1997). Other books by Gordon include:

> *Safety in Numbers: Nurse to Patient Ratios and the Future of Health Care (The Culture and Politics of Health Care Work).* John Buchanan, Tanya Bretherton, and Suzanne Gordon, Cornell University Press, 2008.
>
> *Nursing Against the Odds: How Health Care Cost Cutting, Media Stereotypes and Medical Hubris Undermine Nurses and Patient Care (The Culture and Politics of Health Care Work).* Suzanne Gordon, ILR Press, 2006.
>
> *The Complexities of Care: Nursing Reconsidered (The Culture and Politics of Health Care Work).* Sioban Nelson and Suzanne Gordon, ILP Press, 2006.
>
> *From Silence to Voice: What Nurses Know and Must Communicate to the Public.* Bernice Buresh and Suzanne Gordon, Cornell University Press, 2003.

The Healthcare Industry

Policy and Politics in Nursing and Health Care. Diana Mason, Judith K Leavitt, and Mary Chaffee, Saunders, 2006. Presents a scholarly analysis and narratives from the field to provide an in-depth understanding of such essential issues as lobbying, use of the media, reimbursement, Social Security, Medicare, etc. Especially useful for nurses in leadership roles.

Nurse Case Management in the 21st Century. Edited by Elaine L. Cohen, Mosby Publishing Company, 1996. An outstanding group of essays packed with information about the changing healthcare system with contributions from some of the most knowledgeable and influential nurse leaders and futurists, including Tim Porter-O'Grady.

Reengineering Nursing and Health Care: The Handbook for Organizational Transformation. Suzanne Smith Blancett and Dominick L. Flarey, Aspen Publishers, 1995. This text adapts the framework of the bestselling book

Reengineering the Corporation and applies its principles to understanding how and why healthcare is changing from compartmentalized services to more seamlessly integrated systems. Essential for nurse managers and leadership nurses in general and for all nurses who want an in-depth understanding of the process of hospital and healthcare restructuring.

The Changing World of Work

We Are All Self Employed: The New Social Contract for Working in a Changing World. Cliff Hakim, Berrett-Koehler Publishers, 1994. An excellent guide to shifting from an employee mentality to a self-employed attitude that includes methods of exploring what you want to do, what skills you bring to the marketplace, and who will be most interested in what you have to offer.

To Build the Life You Want, Create the Work You Love: The Spiritual Dimension of Entrepreneuring. Marsha Sinetar, St. Martin's Press, 1995. The sequel to the best selling and widely read book *Do What You Love, The Money Will Follow* will help you create work and/or understand the work you do from an inner-development standpoint in which "your consciousness is the doorway to the answers you want."

Managing at the Speed of Change: How Resilient Managers Succeed and Prosper Where Others Fail. Daryl R. Conner, Villard Books, 1994. Provides a structure and a practical approach to change while dealing with the feelings and behaviors common to the change experience. In addition to explaining what is changing and why in the world of work, this book will assist you in understanding the nature and process of change and translate these into specific strategies for coping effectively with stress.

Beat the Odds: Career Buoyancy Tactics for Today's Turbulent Job Market. Martin Yate, Ballantine Books, 1995. A very readable and useful exploration of how to succeed in the changing world of work. Describes what is changing and why and provides practical suggestions. Topics include why layoffs aren't going to stop and what to do about it; the hot job opportunities, including healthcare; and developing such portable, core career competencies as goal orientation, positive expectancy, inner openness, personal influence, organized action, and informed risk.

C and the Box: A Paradigm Parable. Frank A. Prince, Pfeiffer & Company, 1993. An illustrated story that helps you understand how the conditioning of your past can limit the potential of your future. In an entertaining and creative way, Prince demonstrates the importance of what happens when you get too comfortable with what is familiar.

"The New Deal: What Companies and Employees Owe One Another." Brian O'Reilly, *Fortune*, June 13, 1997. The cover story of this respected business publication explains why loyalty and job security are "nearly dead" and how employers who "deliver honesty and satisfying work can expect a new form of commitment from workers."

Taking Responsibility: Self-Reliance and the Accountable Life. Nathaniel Branden, Simon & Schuster, 1997. An important book for those wishing to broaden and deepen their knowledge of the concept of self-reliance and self-responsibility as it relates to strengthening the self for working and living differently in the 21st century. Written by the psychologist who wrote the classic and best selling book *The Psychology of Self-Esteem.*

Job Shift: How to Prosper in a Workplace Without Jobs. William Bridges, Addison-Wesley, 1995. This book is the source of a *Fortune* magazine cover story, "The End of the Job," and describes how organizations are transforming their employment structure from jobs that represent artificial and overlapping divisions of responsibility to work that needs to be done. Bridges encourages employees to respond to this shift by converting themselves into a business within a market, rather than remain on the payroll of one organization. A clear and concise guide to the facts as well as the psychological impact of "de-jobbing," with specific information about how to run the business you have become, which he calls "You & Co."

"You, Inc.," *U.S. News & World Report,* October 28, 1996. A description of how America has "leapt headlong into the information age, and how careers will never be the same." The historical transition about the way in which work is organized and carried out is outlined, along with career profiles of people who have successfully made the transition to self-managing their careers by becoming "You, Inc., the fastest growing employment segment in the economy."

The Lifetime Career Manager: New Strategies for a New Era. James C. Cabrera and Charles F. Albrecht Jr., Adams, 1995. A comprehensive review of career planning information with a look at how to manage your career without a guarantee of job security. Challenges the myth of cradle-to-grave employment as it provides tips, guidelines, and ideas for shifting to the new employment reality of self-responsibility.

A Manager's Guide to the Millennium: Today's Strategies for Tomorrow's Success. Ken Matejka and Richard J. Dunsing, American Management Association,

1995. An excellent translation of how organizations will look in this new millennium and how to learn the new ground rules to "handle, enjoy, and even shape what's in store for you."

Healing the Wounds: Overcoming the Trauma of Layoffs and Revitalizing the Downsized Organizations. David M. Noer, Jossey-Bass 1993. An indispensable guide to understanding the psychological and interpersonal impact of layoffs on work satisfaction and organizational productivity.

Change, Trends, Predictions, and Statistics

Health and Health Care 2010: The Forecast, The Challenge, 2nd ed. Institute for the Future, Jossey-Bass, 2003. Outlines what's changing in healthcare and why, including trends and predictions related to managed care, the healthcare workforce, remote telemetry, disease management, and more.

Megatrends: 2010. Patricia Aberdeen, Hampton Roads, 2007. Aberdeen builds on John Naisbitt's 1982 classic *Megatrends* book by discussing such 21st-century issues as conscious capitalism, the values-driven consumer, and socially responsible investing. She points out how business is shifting from "greed to enlightened self-interest, from elitism to economic democracy and from the fundamentalist doctrine of 'profit at any cost' to the conscious ideology that espouses both morals and money."

The Tipping Point: How Little Things Can Make a Big Difference. Malcolm Gladwell, Back Bay Books, 2002. A fascinating discussion, chock-full of relevant examples of how epidemics of change are brought about by small, seemingly insignificant events.

Clicking: Sixteen Trends to Future-Fit Your Life, Your Work, and Your Business. Faith Popcorn and Lys Marigold, Harper Collins, 1996. By the futurist and author of the often-quoted Popcorn Report, this book continues the author's ideas and predictions about the business and personal trends that are and will be shaping every aspect of our lives.

Occupational Outlook Handbook. U.S. Department of Labor, Bureau of Labor Statistics, U.S. Government Printing Office, 2008–2009. An essential guide, published annually, to how all occupations have been affected by the dramatic and sweeping changes of the late 20th and the early 21st centuries, including statistics and descriptions of such growth industries as healthcare.

Technology and Nursing Informatics

Informatics and Nursing: Opportunities and Challenges. Linda Q. Thede, Lippincott, Williams & Wilkins, 2003. Excellent coverage of the theories, tools and skills required to understand this emerging nursing specialty, whether you are selecting it as a career option or want a better understanding of the impact of computer communication on healthcare and nursing practice.

Career Management: General Information

What Color Is Your Parachute? 2008: A Practical Manual for Job-Hunters and Career Changers. Richard Nelson Bolles, Ten Speed Press, 2007. Considered by many to be the classic guide and "bible" of career management across all industries, this book is updated annually with a new edition appearing each November. Use this book to identify and utilize your skills more effectively, whether you are job hunting or want to be more marketable in your current place of employment.

I Could Do Anything If I Only Knew What It Was: How to Discover What You Really Want and How to Get It. Barbara Sher, Dell Books, 1995. A guide and sourcebook for overcoming the blocks that prevent you from engaging in the work you want to be doing. This book takes you through a process of self-exploration, including action-oriented goal setting.

Finding a Path with Heart: How to Go from Burnout to Bliss. Beverly Potter, Ronin, 1995. A practical sourcebook that describes how to find work satisfaction and is packed with entertaining and useful drawings, stories, exercises, and quotes.

The Path: Creating Your Mission Statement for Work and for Life. Laurie Beth Jones, Hyperion, 1998. Provides inspiring and practical advice to lead readers through the steps of defining and fulfilling a mission in life. The lessons on creating a mission statement are easily transferable to the world of work.

E-Resumes: Everything You Need to Know about Using Electronic Resumes to Tap into Today's Hot Job Market. Susan Britton Whitcomb and Pat Kendall, McGraw Hill, 2001. An A–Z guide for job seeking in the 21st century with special emphasis on how to construct, post, attach, and send electronic resumes.

Resumes! Resumes! Resumes! 2nd ed. Career Press, 1996. Top career experts from a variety of fields discuss and demonstrate how to compose effective resumes. In addition to information about the art of writing and editing a resume, this book provides many samples from which to style your resume.

Writing That Works: How to Write Effective E-Mails, Letters, Resumes, Presentations, Plans, Reports, and Other Business Communications. Kenneth Roman and Joel Raphaelson, Harper Information, 2000. This book contains especially helpful sections on email and e-writing to ensure professionalism and political correctness.

Nursing-Specific Career Management

"Creating Your Mission Statement for Work and for Life." Paula Schneider, *Nursing Spectrum,* Gannett Satellite Information Network, 1998. Written by a registered nurse who studied with Laurie Beth Jones, author of *The Path: Creating Your Mission Statement for Work and For Life,* this article summarizes the process of creating your mission statement and includes examples of its application to nursing.

What You Need to Know about Today's Workplace: A Survival Guide for Nurses. Lynda Flanagan, American Nurses Publishing, 1996. In addition to explaining how and why the healthcare industry is changing, this book provides useful information about employment rights and protections (such as collective bargaining, at-will employment, and layoffs), employer terms and conditions of employment (such as performance appraisals, grievance handling, and liability protection), and the management of stress and conflicts in restructuring environments. There is an extensive appendix with sources of information on employment rights and protections as well as a comprehensive reference list and bibliography.

Resumes for Nursing Careers. McGraw Hill, 2007. Contains sample resumes and cover letters for nurses, including tips and worksheets to simplify the process.

Nursing Spectrum and Nurse Week Career Fair 2008. Gannett Health Care Group. This excellent career specialty guide is published annually and sent free of charge to nurses who receive *Nursing Spectrum* or *Nurse Week,* also free upon request (log on to *www.nurse.com*). In addition to relevant professional and career articles, this resource provides job listings and career opportunities nationwide.

Reinventing Your Nursing Career: A Handbook for Success in the Age of Managed Care. Michael Newell and Mario Pinardo, Aspen, 1998. Describes how and why nursing and healthcare is changing with special emphasis on managed care opportunities and the healthcare industry as a consumer-driven business environment. Has excellent sections on understanding and developing empowerment.

Career Planning for Nurses. Betty Case, PhD, RN, Delmar, 1997. An informative guide in career management and self-assessment to assist nurses in creating opportunities for blending their strengths with marketplace needs. Contains a special section for student nurses and an excellent chapter on the nurse informatics role.

Self-Care, Stress Management, Work-Life Balance, Personal Growth

Nursing-Specific

Holistic Nursing: A Handbook for Practice, 5th ed. Barbara Montgomery Dossey and Lynn Keegan, Jones and Bartlett, 2008. This is a stress management book disguised as a nursing textbook. Its approaches are useful not only for coping with stress in general but with the particular kind of stress inherent in nursing practice. Packed with information about wellness, the psychophysiology of body-mind healing, nutrition, relaxation strategies, imagery. The authors assist you in consulting the truth within and from that vantage point reaching out more effectively to patients.

Overcoming Secondary Stress in Medical and Nursing Practice: A Guide to Professional and Personal Well-Being. Robert Wicks, Oxford University Press, 2005. Discusses compassion fatigue and burnout. Provides useful self-assessment tools along with strategies for developing a self-care practice.

Transforming Nurses' Stress and Anger: Steps Toward Healing. Sandra Thomas, Springer, 2004. An excellent book on an important topic written in clear and accessible language by a nurse educator and researcher. Offers practical strategies for transforming anger into personal and professional empowerment.

Use Your Anger: A Woman's Guide to Empowerment. Sandra Thomas and Cheryl Jefferson, Pocket Books, 1996. Written by a nurse and based on a seven-year, nationwide study she conducted, this book will help you understand the impact anger may be having on your life and provides you with ways to transform the energy of anger into productive and empowering action.

Healing Yourself: A Nurse's Guide to Self-Care and Renewal. Sherry Kahn and Mileva Saulo, Delmar, 1994. A concise and comprehensive handbook with holistic approaches that are practical and easy to use in order to sustain your "body, mind, and spirit as you meet the daily demands of your challenging career."

Pro-Nurse Handbook: Designed for the Nurse Who Wants to Survive/Thrive Professionally. Melodie Chenevert, Mosby, 1996. An entertaining and useful guide to understanding and managing the personal and interpersonal problems that lead to the loss of work satisfaction and sometimes to burnout. Topics include learning to pace yourself, ways to increase your work satisfaction, dealing with procrastination, and understanding the "business" of nursing.

General

The 7 Habits of Highly Effective People: Powerful Lessons in Personal Change, 15th anniversary ed. Stephen R. Covey, Free Press, 2004. A well-known and widely read classic that presents a "principle-centered" approach for solving professional and personal issues.

First Things First. Stephen R. Covey, A. Roger Merrill, and Rebecca R. Merrill, Free Press, 1996. A time-management book that expands on Covey's time-management approach in *The 7 Habits of Highly Effective People.* Correlates time management with vision, roles, and empowerment principles.

Margin: Restoring Emotional, Physical, Financial, and Time Reserves to Overloaded Lives. Richard A. Swenson, NavPress, 2004. Written by a futurist and physician, this book can help you develop strategies when you have too much to do and too little time to do it.

Take Time for Your Life. Cheryl Richardson, Broadway Books, 2000. Presents strategies for making conscious decisions that affect your life with a section on "extreme self-care."

Minding the Body, Mending the Mind. Joan Borysenko, Da Capo Press, 2007. Written by a psychotherapist and scientist who is described as a pioneer in the new field of psychoneuroimmunology and the founder of the Mind Body Clinic at the New England Deaconess Hospital, this book provides sound and useful information on managing stress as it explains the important relationship between mind and body.

Developing a 21st Century Mind. Marsha Sinetar, Ballentine Books, 1992. This bestselling author of *Do What You Love, the Money Will Follow* describes a process she calls positive structuring, the necessary path to shifting from the traditional mind—which Sinetar argues is fear motivated, dualistic, and egocentric—to the nondualistic and synergistic 21st-century mind needed for living successfully as the world changes. While published in 1992, the principles of this book are current and essential to 21st century living.

Emotional Intelligence: Why It Can Matter More Than IQ. Daniel Goleman, Bantam Books, 1997. This book has become a classic in its field. It presents ground-breaking behavioral research that explains and demonstrates how emotional intelligence is essential to self-awareness, impulse control, self-discipline, persistence, self-motivation, and empathy.

Social Intelligence: Why It Can Matter More Than IQ. Daniel Goleman, Bantam Books, 2007. In this companion to *Emotional Intelligence,* Goleman argues for a new social model based on emerging discoveries in neuorscience. He describes what happens in our brain when we relate to others and how this affects such 21st-century experiences as the use of iPods, multitasking, parenting, and group dynamics.

The Fifth Discipline Fieldbook: Strategies and Tools for Building a Learning Organization. Peter Senge, Currency and Doubleday Books, 1994. A beautifully conceived and organized book based on Senge's classic work, *The Fifth Discipline.* Topics include reinventing relationships, building vision, developing personal mastery, and systems thinking.

Women Who Run with the Wolves: Myths and Stories of the Wild Woman Archetype. Clarissa Pinkola Estes, Ballantine Books, 1996. This book invites you to experience the powerful force within you that is "natural, creative, powerful, filled with good instincts, and ageless knowing." Nurses will especially identify with the chapter called "Homing: Returning to OneSelf."

Revolution from Within: A Book of Self-Esteem. Gloria Steinem, Little, Brown, 1993. An autobiographical account of this feminist's life and journey, primarily from the standpoint of her own personal development, describing the necessary "revolution of spirit and consciousness," which she had always assumed was secondary to social change.

A Passion for the Possible: A Guide to Realizing Your True Potential. Jean Houston, Harper San Francisco, 1998. Creates an understanding of how to break free from the limiting beliefs that will prevent you from taking advantage of the opportunities change always brings.

Self Renewal: High Performance in a High Stress World. Dennis T. Jaffe and Cynthia D. Scott, Crisp, 1995. An extremely useful workbook that contains clear explanations as well as self-assessment tools and self-reflection exercises.

Uses a self-care approach to stress management, presenting ways to increase your self-awareness, self-management, and self-renewal strategies.

The Artist's Way: A Spiritual Path to Higher Creativity. Julia Cameron, Jeremy P. Tarcher, Putnum, 2002. An empowering book to increase the creative expression of any and all areas of your life. Engages you in a 12-week personal development journey to "recover your creativity from a variety of blocks, including limiting beliefs, fear, self-sabotage, jealousy, guilt, addictions, and other inhibiting forces."

Life Skills: Taking Charge of Your Personal and Professional Growth. Richard J. Leider, Pfeiffer, 1999. Takes a personal development viewpoint to career strategies and work success. Life and work planning are explored in an interactive workbook to "help you align your career objectives, talents, and deepest values."

Changing for Good: The Revolutionary Program That Explains the Six Stages of Change and Teaches You How to Free Yourself from Bad Habits. James Prochaska, John Norcross, Carlo Di Clemente, William Morrow and Co., 1996. A well-organized approach to change with some refreshing reinterpretations that demystify the process and provide clear strategies for effective coping.

Resilience: How to Bounce Back When the Going Gets Tough. Frederic Flach, Hatherleigh Press, 1998. A simple stress management guide with easy-to-understand descriptions of how stress happens and how to handle it. Topics include the response to stress at different points in the life cycle, what the resilient personality looks like, and how self-worth is related to resilience.

Thriving in Transition: Effective Living in Times of Change. Marcia Perkins-Reed, Touchstone Books, 1996. An easy-to-read and extremely useful book that takes a holistic approach to adapting to change, using information from the fields of psychology, organizational development, physics, and spirituality.

The Dance of Anger: A Woman's Guide to Changing the Patterns of Intimate Relationships. Harriet Lerner, Harper, 1997. A classic and perennially useful book, packed with examples and suggestions, which discusses why anger is misunderstood and culturally reinforced with negative stereotypes, eventually robbing women (and men as well) of autonomy and power in relationships.

Retirement Readiness

Encore: Finding Work That Matters in the Second Half of Life. Marc Freedman, Public Affairs, 2007. Freedman provides inspirational and factual arguments for baby boomers considering whether to continue working and, if so, how. Contains many profiles of people who are benefiting from what he calls the "encore society," including Jacqueline Khan, a 64-year-old critical care nurse.

Prime Time: How Baby Boomers Will Revolutionize Retirement and Transform America. Marc Freedman, Public Affairs, 2000. In *Prime Time,* Freedman, who also wrote *Encore,* writes about how baby boomers will become social activists and rewrite the retirement rules because they "will not accept the old notions of later life." Additional discussions include his ideas about what businesses and government need to do to keep this valuable human resource in the workforce and the benefits of doing so.

Age Wave: How the Most Important Trend of Our Time Can Change Your Future. Ken Dychtwald and Joe Flower, Bantam Books,1990. Written by a psychologist and gerontologist, *Age Wave* is packed with important data and descriptions of changing behavioral patterns, including trends in work, lifestyles, and personal relationships. Dychtwald forecasts how these changes in the baby boom generation will affect how we think and live.

Index

INDEX

F–G

H

I

K–L

M

N

O–P

R

610.730699 VALLANO
Vallano, Annette
Your career in nursing

R0119654922 EAST_A

EAST ATLANTA
Atlanta-Fulton Public Library